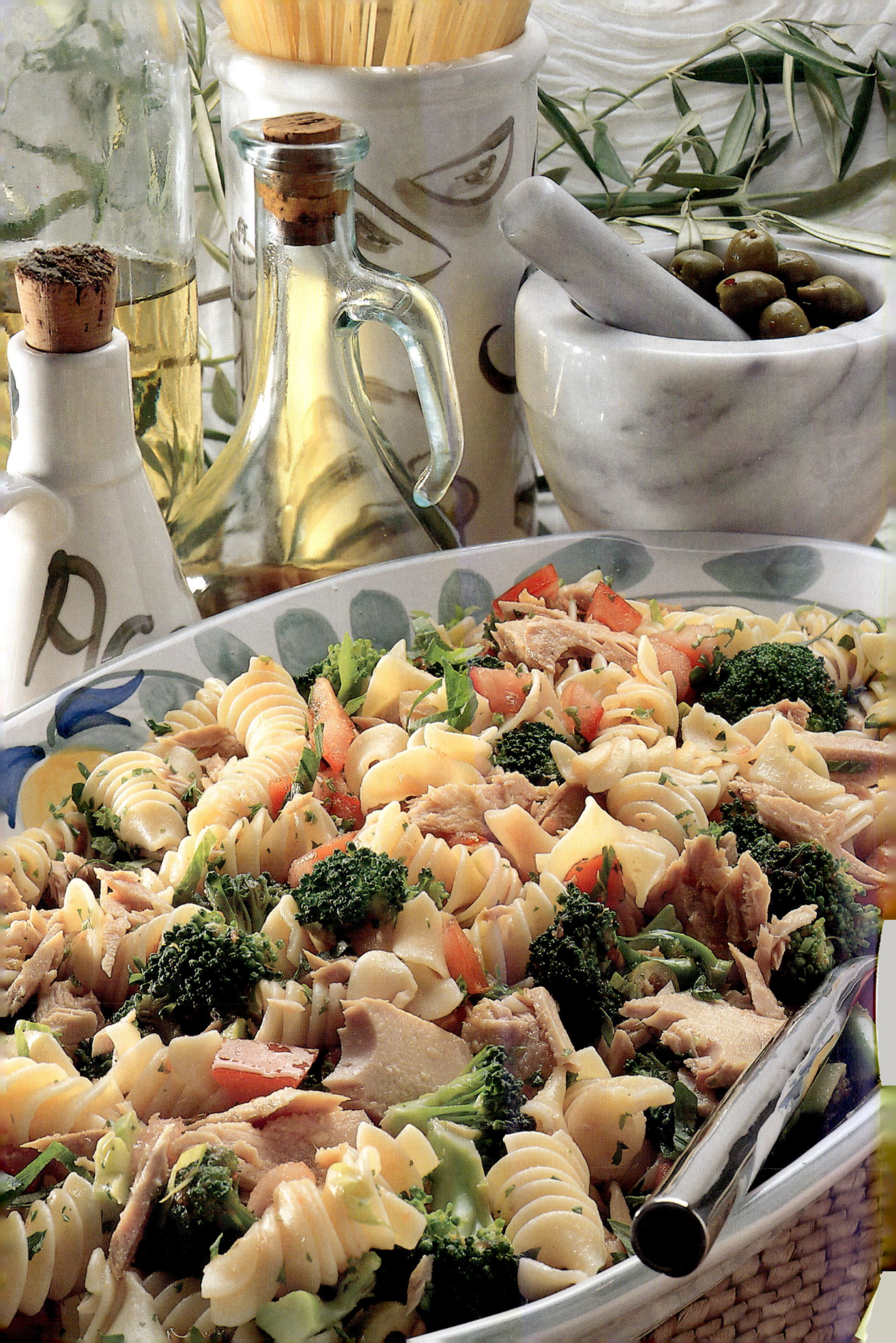

WEIGHT WATCHERS®

Quick & Easy Cookbook

WEIGHT WATCHERS®

Quick & Easy Cookbook

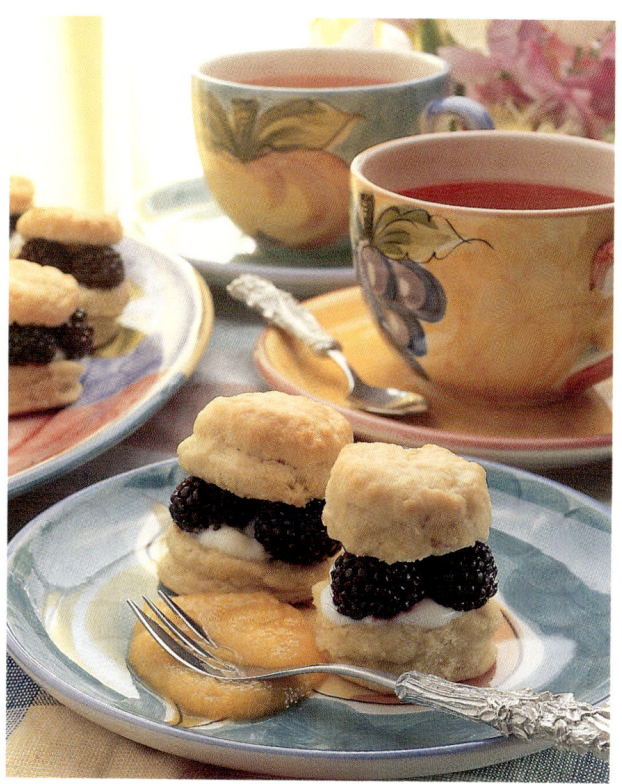

COMPASS PUBLISHING CO. PTY. LIMITED

2nd Floor, 44 Miller Street, North Sydney, NSW, 2060, Australia

Retail edition distributed exclusively by

PENGUIN BOOKS AUSTRALIA LTD,

487 Maroondah Highway, Ringwood, Victoria, 3134, Australia

Recipe development and food styling: Allyson Gofton
Nutrition consultant: Rosemary Stanton
Technical analysis: Meaghan Stanton
Photography: Alan Gillard

Published by Compass Publishing Co. Pty. Limited,
2nd Floor, 44 Miller Street, North Sydney, NSW, 2060, Australia
Tel: (02) 9955 2777 Fax: (02) 9955 2333
New Zealand Office: (09) 262 2314

First published 1995

Retail edition distributed exclusively by Penguin Books Australia Ltd,
487 Maroondah Highway, Ringwood, Victoria, 3134, Australia

10 9 8 7 6 5 4 3 2 1

National Library of Australia
Cataloguing-in-Publication data

  Weight Watchers quick & easy cookbook.

  Includes index.
  ISBN 0 670 86587 7.

  1. Low-calorie diet – Recipes. 2. Reducing diets –
  Recipes. 3. Quick and easy cookery. I. Weight Watchers
  International. II. Title: Quick and easy cookbook.

  641.5635

Typeset by ACP Colour Graphics Pty. Ltd., Sydney, NSW, Australia
Printed in Australia by Griffin Press Limited

Weight Watchers and *Weight Watchers* are registered
trademarks of Weight Watchers International, Inc.

Pictured on front cover: *Strawberries in Wine Jelly (page 98) and Jaffaberry Sherbet (page 100).*
Pictured on back cover, clockwise from top: *Steak and Crispy Potato Cakes (page 64); Seafood Tacos (page 16); Pasta with Brie and Green Beans (page 86); Chicken Jalouise (page 46).*
Pictured on page 2, *Tuna on Pasta (recipe page 24);* **Pictured page 3,** *Fruit Shortcakes (recipe page 94);* **Pictured page 6,** *Snacks (recipes start page 114).*

Publisher's Note

Welcome to this fabulous new addition to the Weight Watchers range of cookery books — *Quick & Easy* — which is packed with delicious meals that will help you lose weight while still eating the foods you enjoy.

The recipes, specially developed for Weight Watchers and based on the successful Weight Watchers Program, are designed to give quick, positive results and are suitable for members and non-members alike.

We have taken the guesswork out of good nutrition and, for the first time, included the Fat and Dietary Fibre content of each recipe to assist those following the latest Weight Watchers Eating Plan. There are dozens of delicious dishes, each made to serve four, so that you can plan well-balanced meals for all the family.

The recipes have been double-tested and include microwave alternatives where possible for your favourites, from seafood, chicken and meat, vegetarian to mouth-watering desserts. We've also included useful serving suggestions and variations, handy hints and cooking tips.

Creating this Weight Watchers cookbook took a great deal of dedication and hard work. For this, we must thank Allyson Gofton* for developing the recipes; the staff of the Weight Watchers New Zealand Auckland office, in particular Liz McCarthy; well-known Australian nutritionist Rosemary Stanton, for her guidance and advice on nutritional aspects of the Weight Watchers Program and Meaghan Stanton for providing nutritional data.

We thank them all for bringing their special skills and enthusiasm to this book.

* Allyson Gofton is an Australian now resident in New Zealand. Originally from Tasmania, Allyson first trained as a chef before continuing her studies in London at Leith's School of Food and Wine. From there she moved to New Zealand to live and worked for the *New Zealand Women's Weekly* for four years before working in the USA and UK with Galloping Gourmet Graham Kerr. Allyson is the Food Editor of New Zealand's leading women's monthly magazine, *NEXT,* and has published three books under her own name, also available in Australia. This is her second book for Weight Watchers.

Contents

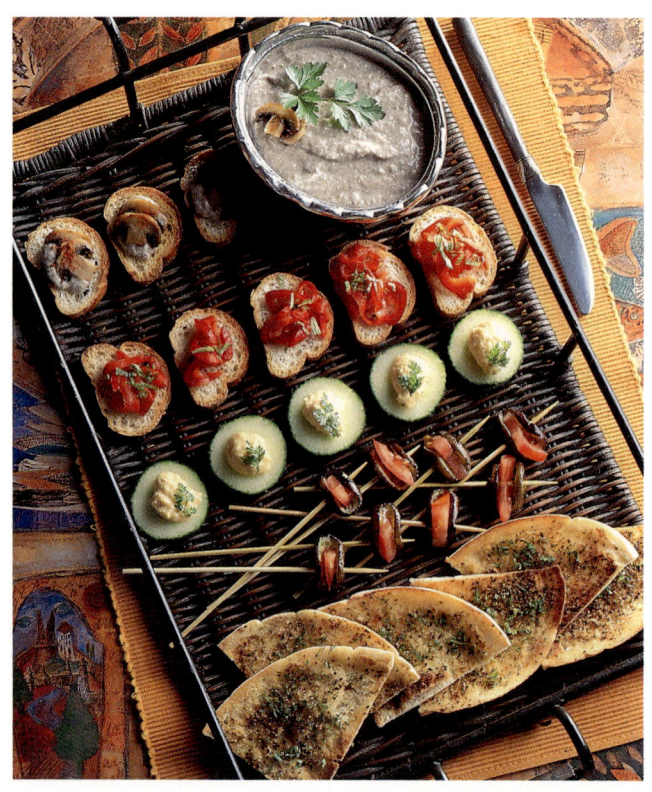

About Our Recipes

The Weight Watchers weight-loss program has been developed to provide as much flexibility and variety in food and recipes as is possible. These easy-to-prepare recipes reflect our changing tastes and eating habits and have been designed to give positive results for those on the Weight Watchers Program.

Members attending meetings will know that the Weight Watchers Program is based on the Selection Information system. Basically, Selections are food servings of similar nutrient content.

▶ Each recipe in this cookbook is followed by a Selection Information statement which tells you how one serving prepared from that recipe fits the Food Plan. If you make any changes in the recipes, please be sure to adjust the Selection information per serving accordingly.

▶ Each recipe gives the Selections for Fruit, Vegetables, Fat, Protein, Bread, Milk and Optional Kilojoules.

▶ The Fat and Dietary Fibre count are also given for each recipe to help those members following the most up-to-date Weight Watchers Program.

▶ Photographed recipes may vary as to the number of servings shown. Please see recipes for exact serving information.

A NOTE ON MICROWAVE COOKING

The recipes in this book were tested in a 700 watt microwave oven. The cooking times given can only be used as a guide as they will vary due to so many factors – the temperature of the food when it is placed in the microwave, the wattage of your oven (check your manual) and the thickness and cut of the meats and vegetables.

METHOD

The method and manner in which the recipes have been developed should be noted by Weight Watchers members.

▶ In any recipe of more than one serving, it is important to mix the ingredients well and divide the mixture evenly to ensure that every portion has an equal amount of each ingredient.

▶ Where liquid and solid parts have to be divided evenly when serving, first drain the liquid, set it aside and divide the remaining ingredients equally; add equal amounts of the liquid to each portion.

FATS & OILS

When vegetable oil is called for, oils such as safflower, sunflower, soybean, corn, cottonseed or any combination of these may be used. In some recipes olive oil and sesame oil, because of their distinctive flavours, have been specifically indicated.

To reduce the amount of fat used in cooking and therefore reduce the kilojoule intake, lightly coat cookware with non-stick cooking spray. We have used non-stick pans where possible throughout this book.

WEIGHING

It is important to weigh and measure ingredients accurately to achieve the best results; this is vital to both recipe results and weight control.

▶ The recipes in this book were developed using Australian Standard Measures, thus one teaspoon equals 5mL and one tablespoon is equal to four teaspoons, 20mL. In New Zealand, one tablespoon is equal to three teaspoons, 15mL.

▶ Always use accurate spoon and cup measures and a scale to weigh foods.

▶ To measure liquids, use a standard glass or clear plastic measuring cup. Always read the markings at eye level and make sure the container is placed on a level surface before you take the reading. To measure less than $\frac{1}{4}$ cup, use standard measuring spoons, available in sets.

▶ To measure dry ingredients, use metal or plastic measuring cups that come in sets of four: $\frac{1}{4}$ cup, $\frac{1}{3}$ cup, $\frac{1}{2}$ cup and 1 cup. Spoon the ingredients into the cup, then level with the straight edge of a knife or metal spatula. To measure less than $\frac{1}{4}$ cup, use standard measuring spoons and, unless directed otherwise, level as you would a measuring cup.

HERBS & SPICES

We have specified the use of mainly fresh herbs in our recipes, however, dried may be substituted. If you are substituting dried herbs for fresh, use approximately $\frac{1}{4}$ the amount of fresh (for example, $\frac{1}{4}$ teaspoon dried basil instead of 1 teaspoon chopped fresh basil). If dried herbs are indicated and you wish to substitute fresh, use approximately four times the amount of dried (1 teaspoon chopped fresh parsley instead of $\frac{1}{4}$ teaspoon dried parsley leaves). If you are substituting ground (powdered) herbs for dried leaves, use approximately half the amount of dried ($\frac{1}{4}$ teaspoon ground thyme instead of $\frac{1}{2}$ teaspoon dried thyme leaves).

▶ If you are substituting fresh spices for ground, use approximately eight times the amount of ground (for example, 1 teaspoon grated fresh ginger instead of $\frac{1}{8}$ teaspoon ground ginger).

▶ Generally, dried herbs and spices should not be kept for more than a year. Usually, if the herb or spice is aromatic, it is still potent.

THE RECIPES

Some of our recipes may make use of certain unusual ingredients. Don't be afraid to explore and experiment with these foods as they will add exciting new flavours to your cooking. All the ingredients featured in the recipes in this book are available in Australia and New Zealand.

▶ Unless otherwise specified, fresh fruit has been used in recipes, but frozen or canned fruit packed in natural juice, with no sugar added, may be substituted.

▶ We have used fresh vegetables unless otherwise indicated. If you choose to substitute the frozen or canned varieties, it may be necessary to adjust the cooking time.

▶ Always buy the leanest meat possible. It is often best to buy meat, remove any visible fat and mince it yourself to avoid fatty mince. Meat and poultry skin should be removed, whenever possible, before cooking.

▶ Small Maggi stock cubes were used in our recipe development and testing. An allowance of 1 small cube or 1 teaspoon of stock powder per 1 cup (250mL) of water has been calculated and counted as 50 Optional Kilojoules. If you are using larger stock cubes adjust the Selection information per serving accordingly.

▶ All the recipes in this cookbook have been developed without any additional salt. If you are accustomed to cooking with salt, try lemon juice as an alternative, squeezed just prior to serving.

▶ Where a recipe calls for drained canned tuna please note that we have selected tuna packed in brine or spring water, not in oil.

▶ Use only low-fat yoghurt in natural or reduced-kilojoule flavours as specified in the recipe ingredients lists.

TIPS FOR BEST RESULTS

When trying a recipe for the first time, take a few minutes to read through the ingredients and directions. By doing this you will know everything you require and exactly what you have to do to prepare the dish successfully.

▶ Always preheat the oven; the time this will take will vary depending on the appliance. We have not included instructions to preheat the oven at the beginning of each recipe. Keep this in mind when using the oven and make sure the required temperature has been reached by the time you are ready to place the dish in the oven. The usual time to preheat an oven varies from 15 to 20 minutes.

▶ The cooking times on most recipes are approximate and should be used as guides. Remember, not all ovens are alike, so be sure to check that the dish is cooked as directed in the recipe.

▶ Avoid marinating foods in aluminium containers. Certain foods react with aluminium and this can have an adverse effect. Rather, glass or stainless-steel containers should be used.

▶ Mussels should be purchased fresh and should have shells that are tightly closed. Give any slightly open shells a hard tap and they should snap shut, but if they don't, do not use them. Remember that shells will open during cooking; any that remain closed should be discarded. It is a good idea to buy more shellfish than you need for the recipe in case you need to discard some, but only serve the quantity specified in the recipe.

FROM THE SEA

Fish is one of our finest foods, as economical as any meat. We should include it regularly in our diets, preferably twice a week. It takes very little time to prepare and is available in many varieties all year round. Use your fishmonger: he is there not only to sell seafood, but to scale, fillet and clean it. If your supermarket sells fish, make sure it has reached the shelves that day. Always cook fish the day you buy it. All seafood is very perishable and does not freeze well.

Spanish Squid

2 teaspoons olive oil

3 cloves garlic, crushed

1 teaspoon paprika

2 cups chopped canned tomatoes in juice

$^1/_2$ cup chopped fresh parsley

2 cups fish stock

600g squid tubes or preferred fish

Pepper to season

1 Heat the oil in a saucepan and cook the garlic and paprika over a low heat for 2 to 3 minutes until the garlic begins to soften.

2 Add the tomatoes and mash well. Stir in the parsley and fish stock and simmer for about 10 minutes.

3 Cut the squid tubes open. Place what would have been the inside of each squid tube on a chopping board. Using a sharp knife, slash the squid diagonally. Do not cut right through the tubes but mark into 2cm square pieces.

4 Add these pieces to the tomato mixture and simmer for 5 minutes. Season well with pepper.

Cook's Tip

▶ To serve ladle the stew into four bowls with rice in the bottom of each. Allow 1 cup cooked rice (hot) per person.

SERVES 4

Each serve provides:
1 Vegetable, $^1/_2$ Fat,
2 Protein,
25 Optional Kilojoules.
Per serve:
5g Fat, $2^1/_2$g Dietary Fibre.

Spanish Squid.

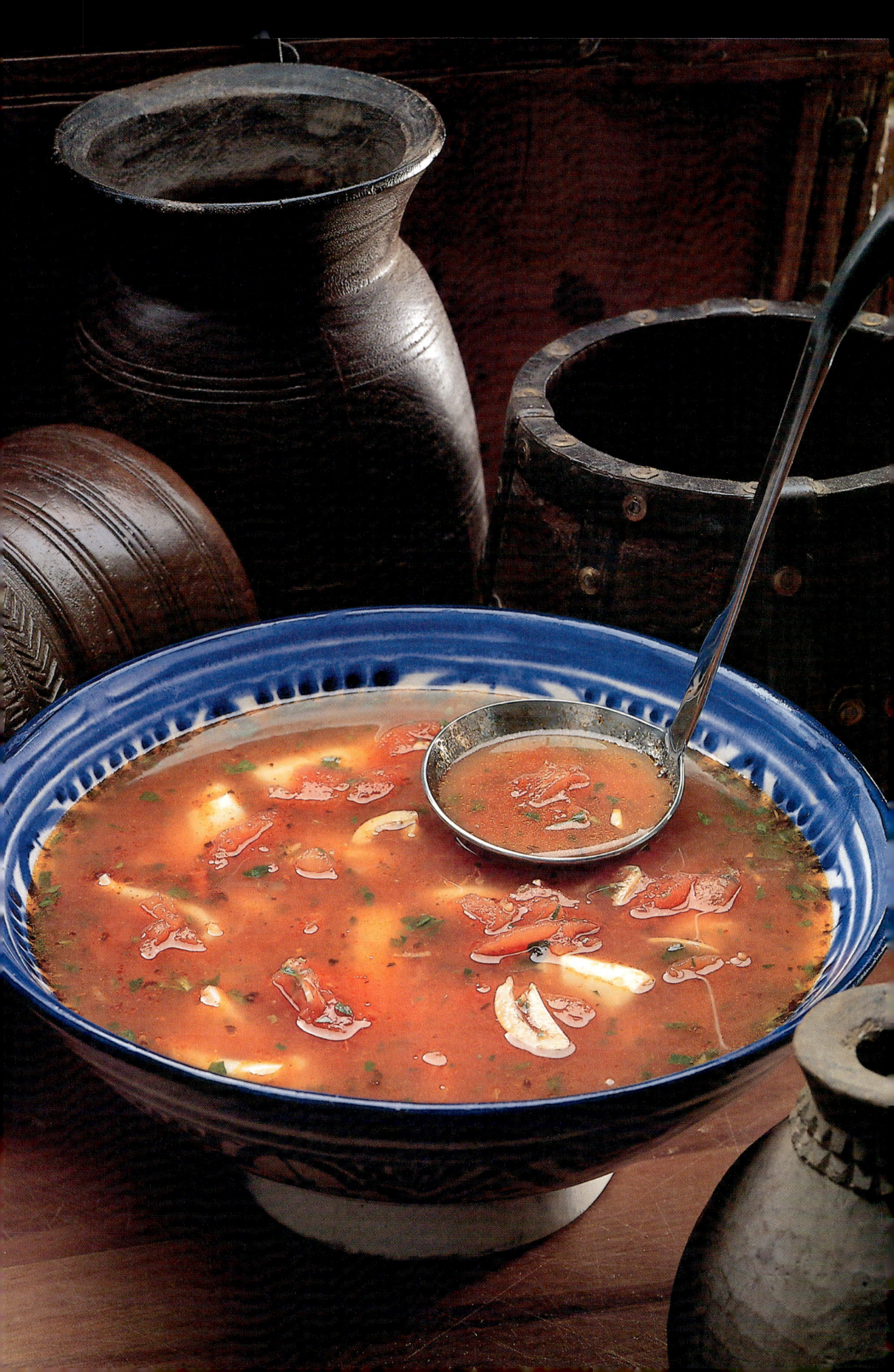

Mussels with Fennel

24 fresh mussels in shell

1 cup fish or vegetable stock

2 cloves garlic, crushed but not peeled

Few black peppercorns

$\frac{1}{2}$ onion, halved and not peeled

1 teaspoon olive oil

1 cup finely chopped onion

$\frac{1}{2}$ cup sliced fennel bulb

$\frac{1}{4}$ cup tomato paste

2 cups chopped fresh tomatoes

1 teaspoon cornflour

2 tablespoons chopped feathery fennel fronds

Pepper to season

4x60g pita bread

1. Scrub the mussels well and pull away the beards, discarding any mussels that are open.

2. Put the stock, garlic, peppercorns and halved onion into a pan and bring to a rapid boil. Add the mussels all at once. Cover and cook over a high heat for 3 to 5 minutes until all the shells have opened. Discard any that do not open.

3. Remove the mussels from their shells and weigh the meat. You will need 480g. Strain and reserve the cooking liquid. Cut the mussels into two or three pieces and set aside.

4. Heat the olive oil in a frying pan and add the onion and fennel. Cook until the onion is soft but not brown.

5. Stir in the tomato paste and cook until slightly darkened. Add the tomatoes and reserved cooking liquid, and simmer for 1 to 2 minutes. Stir the cornflour to a paste with a splash of water and stir into the tomato mixture. Simmer for 1 to 2 minutes.

6. Add the mussels and chopped fennel and season well with pepper. Serve immediately with pita bread.

Cook's Tips

▶ Buy several extra mussels as any that do not open during cooking must be discarded. Mussels should be cooked on the day they are purchased.

▶ This dish can also be served with rice or pasta.

SERVES 4

EACH SERVE PROVIDES:
2 Vegetable, $\frac{1}{4}$ Fat,
2 Protein, 2 Bread,
25 Optional Kilojoules.
PER SERVE:
$5\frac{1}{2}$g Fat, $4\frac{1}{2}$g Dietary Fibre.

Salmon Mousse

4 teaspoons poly-unsaturated margarine

1¹/₂ tablespoons plain flour

1 cup fish stock

50g light cream cheese

¹/₂ cup minced spring onions

¹/₄ cup lemon juice

2 tablespoons chopped fresh dill or parsley

1 teaspoon Dijon mustard

3 teaspoons gelatine

¹/₄ cup water

240g cooked fresh salmon, flaked

2 egg whites

1. Melt the margarine in a saucepan. Add the flour and cook for about 1 minute until frothy. Remove from the heat and stir in the stock. Return to the heat and continue to stir until the sauce thickens.

2. Add the cheese, spring onions, lemon juice, chopped dill and mustard. Set aside to cool.

3. Add the gelatine to the water and leave to swell. Dissolve over hot water or place in the microwave and heat on 100% power for 10 to 15 seconds.

4. Blend or process the sauce, gelatine and flaked salmon until smooth. Transfer to a bowl and refrigerate until almost set.

5. Whip the egg whites in a clean bowl until thick. Fold into the salmon mixture gently.

6. Pour into a wetted 3-cup capacity mould and refrigerate for 4 hours or until set. Turn out and slice to serve.

Variations

▶ If you do not have fish stock, use vegetable stock or milk, and alter your Selections accordingly.

▶ The salmon can be grilled or poached. You can substitute fresh salmon with canned salmon or tuna.

Cook's Tip

▶ Serve the mousse with salad or as an entrée.

SERVES 4

EACH SERVE PROVIDES:
¹/₄ Vegetable, 1 Fat,
1 Protein,
210 Optional Kilojoules.
PER SERVE:
10g Fat, ¹/₂g Dietary Fibre.

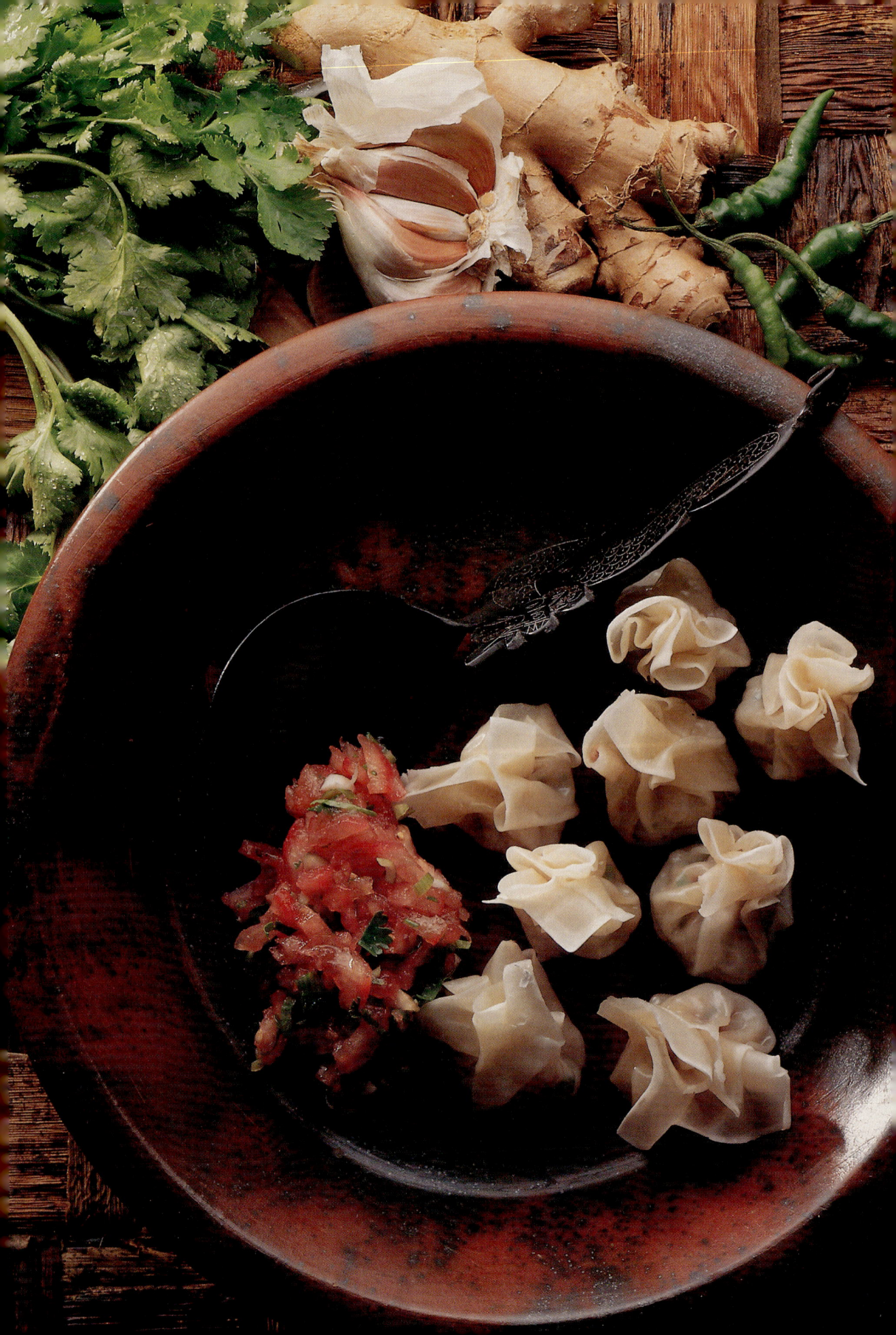

Wontons with Tomato Salsa

WONTONS

1 teaspoon sesame oil

1 teaspoon each crushed garlic and chopped fresh ginger

1/2 cup chopped spring onions

160g lean minced pork

240g shelled and deveined cooked prawns or shrimps, finely diced

3 teaspoons hoisin sauce

2 egg whites

150g drained water chestnuts, finely chopped

32 wonton wrappers (10cm square) about 60g per person

TOMATO SALSA

3 cups diced tomatoes

1/4 cup chopped spring onions

1 green chilli, seeded and chopped

1/4 cup chopped fresh coriander

1 tablespoon white vinegar

Pepper to season

1. To prepare the wontons, heat the oil in a frying pan and cook the garlic, ginger and spring onions for 1 minute. Alternatively, cook the oil, garlic, ginger and spring onions in a covered microwave-safe container for 1 minute on 100% power. Leave to cool.

2. In a bowl, combine this mixture with the pork mince, prawns, hoisin sauce, egg whites and water chestnuts.

3. Take one wonton wrapper in your hand and brush with water. Place a small spoonful of mixture in the centre and bring the edges together to form a parcel, squeezing the dough just above the meat filling.

4. Repeat this process with remaining mixture and wrappers to make 32 wontons.

5. Arrange the wontons in a bamboo steamer or stacked steamers. Place over a pot of rapidly boiling water and steam for 6 to 7 minutes until the wontons are cooked. Serve with the salsa.

6. To prepare the salsa, blend or process the tomatoes, spring onions, chilli, coriander and vinegar. Pulse to a coarse texture. Season with pepper and mix well.

Cook's Tip

▶ Enjoy these wontons with rice and vegetables, stir-fried with ginger and garlic.

SERVES 4

EACH SERVE PROVIDES:
2 Vegetable, 1/4 Fat,
2 Protein, 2 1/2 Bread,
65 Optional Kilojoules.
PER SERVE:
3 1/2 g Fat, 4g Dietary Fibre.

Wontons with Tomato Salsa.

Seafood Tacos

4 taco shells

1½ cups shredded lettuce

SEAFOOD SAUCE

2 cups chopped fresh tomatoes

½ cup chopped spring onions

1 clove garlic, crushed

¼ cup tomato juice

1–2 tablespoons chopped mild jalapeño peppers

1 tablespoon each chopped fresh coriander and parsley

¼–½ teaspoon each ground coriander and cumin

300g mixed seafood e.g. diced fresh fish, prawns, surimi, squid

REFRIED BEANS

240g cooked pinto beans

¼ cup evaporated skim milk

2 tablespoons tomato paste

¼ teaspoon each ground coriander and cumin

½ cup chicken stock

Pepper to season

SERVES 4

EACH SERVE PROVIDES:
2 Vegetable, 2 Protein,
1 Bread,
60 Optional Kilojoules.
PER SERVE:
5g Fat, 7g Dietary Fibre.

1 To prepare the sauce, put the tomatoes, spring onions, garlic, tomato juice, jalapeño peppers, fresh coriander and parsley, ground coriander and cumin into a small frying pan and simmer for 3 to 4 minutes.

2 Add the seafood and simmer for 4 to 5 minutes until the seafood is cooked.

3 To make the refried beans, mash the cooked pinto beans in a pan until smooth. Stir in the evaporated milk, tomato paste and spices, and mix to a paste.

4 Heat through. Stir in chicken stock and reheat. Season with pepper.

5 Heat the taco shells, fill with lettuce, refried beans and seafood sauce. Serve hot.

Microwave Method

1 To prepare the sauce, put the tomatoes, spring onions, garlic, tomato juice and jalapeño peppers in a shallow microwave-safe dish. Cover with plastic or a lid and cook on 100% power for 5 minutes.

2 Add the fresh coriander and parsley, ground coriander and cumin and seafood. Cover and cook on 70% power for 5 to 6 minutes until the seafood is almost cooked. Leave for 1 minute.

3 To make the refried beans, mash the cooked pinto beans until smooth. Stir in the evaporated milk, tomato paste and spices, and mix to a paste.

4 Cover and cook on 100% power for 3 to 4 minutes until hot. Stir in stock and heat. Season with pepper.

5 Heat the taco shells, fill with lettuce, refried beans and seafood sauce. Serve hot.

Cook's Tip

▶ Accompany with summer vegetables, such as tomatoes and cucumber.

Seafood Tacos.

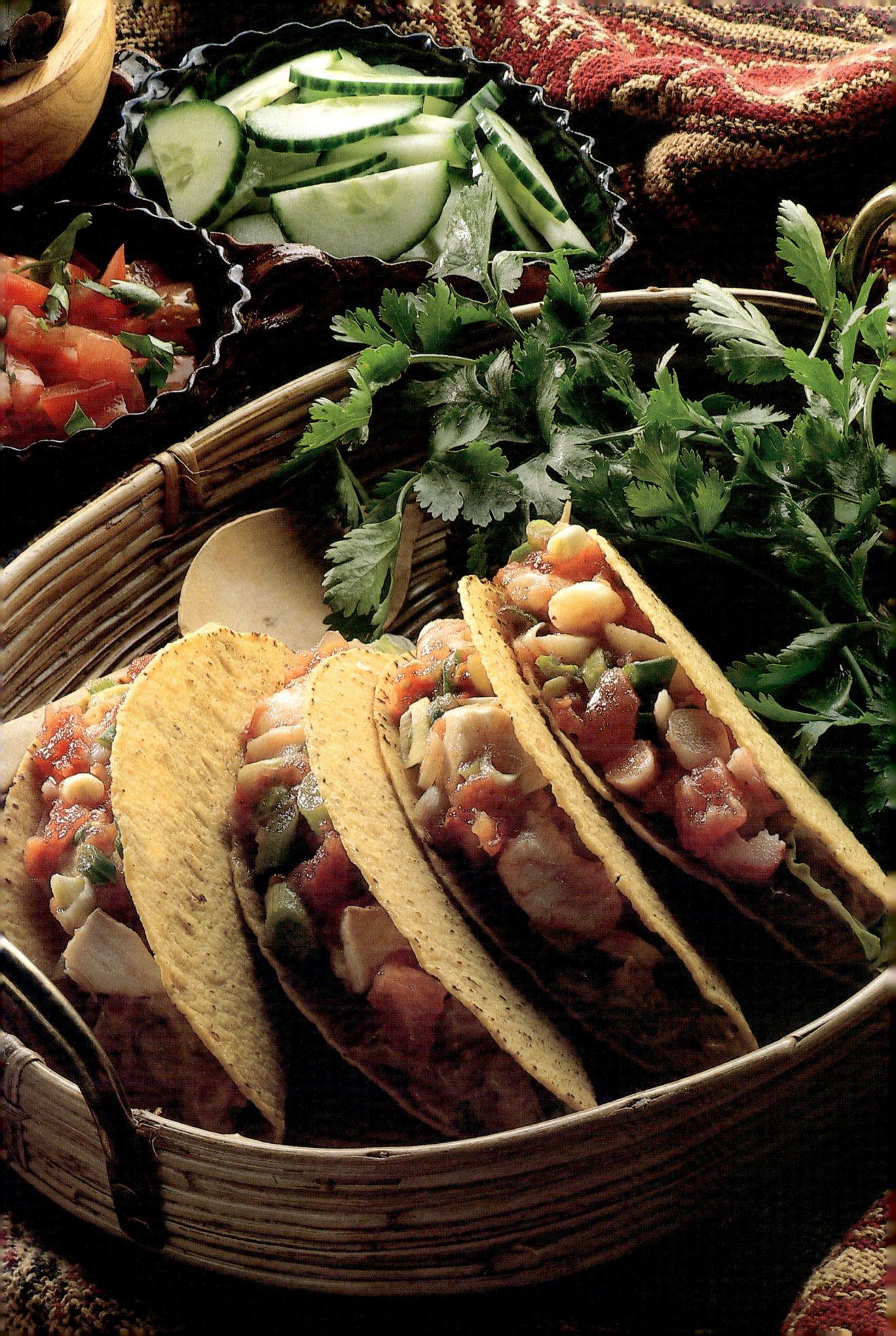

Tuna and Potato Slice

1 medium
red capsicum

600g cooked whole
potatoes, cold

¹/₄ cup chopped parsley

¹/₂ cup sliced
spring onions

1 egg, beaten

3 teaspoons
mustard pickles

2 tablespoons
chopped fresh dill

180g canned tuna,
drained and flaked

1 Heat the oven to 240°C and cook the capsicum for 15 to 20 minutes until it is blackened all over. Leave to cool in a freezer bag, then peel away the charred skin and remove the core and seeds. Slice very finely and set aside.

2 Grate the potatoes into a bowl and combine with the parsley, spring onions, beaten egg, pickles and dill, mixing together well.

3 Spread half the mixture in a lightly greased 18cm or 20cm springform cake tin. Top with the flaked tuna and sliced capsicum, then cover with the second half of the potato, pressing firmly with a fork.

4 Bake at 200°C for 20 to 25 minutes until hot and golden. Serve warm.

Cook's Tip

▶ This recipe is quick to prepare and makes use of leftover potatoes – also leftover cold fish, canned or fresh salmon or smoked fish.

SERVES 4

EACH SERVE PROVIDES:
1 Vegetable, 1 Protein,
1¹/₂ Bread,
20 Optional Kilojoules.
PER SERVE:
3g Fat, 2¹/₂g Dietary Fibre.

Salmon Roulade

1¼ cups skim milk

1 tablespoon cornflour

¼ cup finely sliced spring onions

3 tablespoons chopped fresh dill, parsley or chives

3 eggs, separated

FILLING

60g quark or cottage cheese

3 teaspoons lemon juice

2 teaspoons chopped capers

240g canned salmon, drained and flaked

¾ cup peeled, diced cucumber

1. Heat 1 cup milk to scalding point. Blend the remaining milk with the cornflour and stir into the hot milk. Cook over a low heat until it thickens. Alternatively, heat 1 cup milk in a microwave-safe bowl on 100% power for 2 minutes. Mix the remaining milk and cornflour, stir in and cook on 100% power for 2 to 3 minutes, stirring occasionally until thick.

2. Mix the spring onions, dill and egg yolks into the cornflour sauce. Beat the egg whites in a clean bowl until stiff and fold into the sauce.

3. Pour the mixture into a paper-lined and greased 33x23cm Swiss roll tin. Bake at 200°C for 10 to 12 minutes until firm to the touch. Turn out onto a clean tea-towel.

4. To prepare the filling, blend the quark, lemon juice, capers, salmon and cucumber.

5. Spread the base with the filling, leaving a 1cm border around the edge. Roll up from the bottom, using the tea-towel as a guide. Serve the roulade hot or cold.

Cook's Tip

▶ Accompany this dish with salad greens and fresh bread.

SERVES 4

EACH SERVE PROVIDES:
½ Vegetable,
2 Protein, ¼ Milk,
75 Optional Kilojoules.
PER SERVE:
10g Fat, ½g Dietary Fibre.

Minted Salmon Fish Cakes

900g peeled potatoes

1¹⁄₂ cups finely chopped leeks

3 tablespoons water

360g canned salmon, drained and flaked

1¹⁄₂ tablespoons chopped fresh mint

2 teaspoons horseradish sauce

Freshly ground black pepper to season

40g dried breadcrumbs

20g grated fresh Parmesan cheese (optional)

1 tablespoon chopped fresh mint

1 Cook the potatoes in boiling water until tender. Drain and mash until smooth.

2 Toss the leeks and water in a frying pan, stirring constantly over a moderate heat for 4 minutes, until cooked. Alternatively, put the leeks and water in a microwave-safe dish and cook on 100% power for 4 minutes until the leeks soften.

3 In a bowl, mix the mashed potatoes, leeks, flaked salmon, 1¹⁄₂ tablespoons mint, horseradish sauce and pepper to season. Divide into eight equal portions.

4 Blend the breadcrumbs, Parmesan and mint and sprinkle on a large plate. Mould the fish servings into eight even shaped cakes and press into the crumb mixture.

5 Bake the fish cakes on a lightly greased oven tray at 190°C for 15 minutes. Turn the fish cakes over and cook for a further 5 to 7 minutes until hot.

NOTE: If omitting the Parmesan cheese, reduce Optional Kilojoules per serve to 80.

Variation

▶ This recipe tastes great with flaked cooked fish or canned tuna. You could also try minced smoked chicken.

Cook's Tip

▶ Serve with vegetables or salad.

SERVES 4

WITH 2 CAKES PER PERSON.
EACH SERVE PROVIDES:
1 Vegetable,
1¹⁄₂ Protein, 2¹⁄₂ Bread,
160 Optional Kilojoules.
PER SERVE:
7g Fat, 6¹⁄₂g Dietary Fibre.

Minted Salmon Fish Cakes served with salad greens.

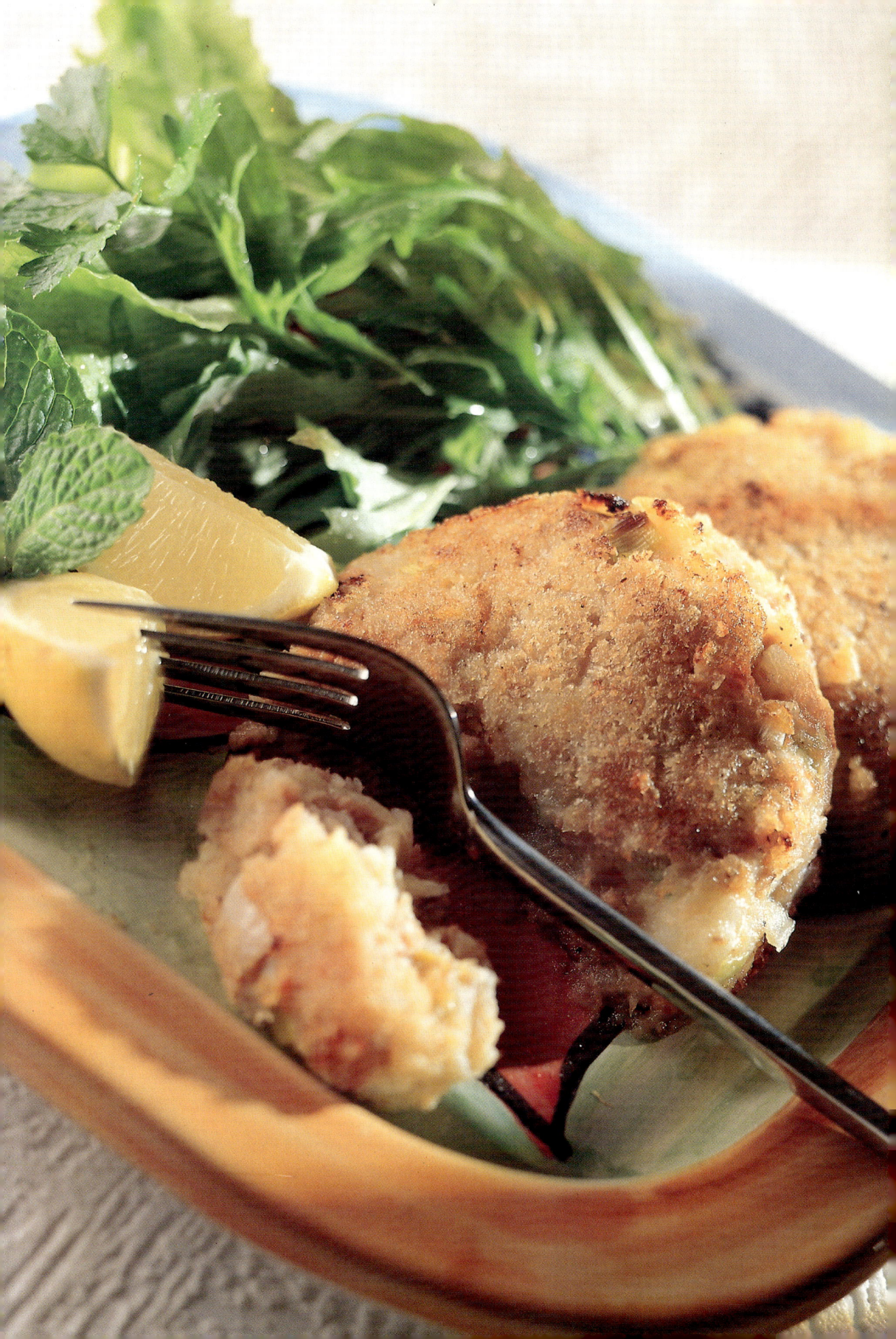

Stuffed Eggplant

2 small eggplants
(about 300g each)

1 teaspoon salt

Fresh basil leaves
to garnish

FILLING

1 teaspoon olive oil

3 cloves garlic, crushed

2 cups diced green
capsicum

$^1/_2$ cup tomato paste

2 cups diced
fresh tomatoes

$^1/_2$ cup chopped
spring onions

2 tablespoons chopped
fresh basil

360g canned tuna
in water, drained
and flaked

Ground black pepper
to season

1. Remove the stems from the eggplants and slice them in half lengthways. Scoop out the flesh to within 1cm of the edge and set aside. Sprinkle the hollowed out shells with the salt and stand for 30 minutes. Rinse well and pat dry.

2. Bake the eggplant shells at 180°C for 15 minutes.

3. To prepare the filling, heat the oil in a frying pan and cook the garlic and capsicum for about 3 minutes. Add the tomato paste and stir over a moderate heat for a further 3 minutes until the sauce darkens a little.

4. Chop and add the eggplant pulp, tomatoes, spring onions and basil. Simmer for 5 minutes until the mixture thickens. Stir in the flaked tuna and season with pepper.

5. Divide the mixture between the eggplant halves. Return to the oven and cook for a further 30 minutes at 180°C until tender. Serve hot, garnished with basil.

Microwave Method

1. Follow the recipe steps 1 and 2.

2. To prepare the filling, cook the garlic and capsicum with a splash of water in a covered microwave-safe container on 100% power for 2 minutes.

3. Add the eggplant pulp, tomato paste, tomatoes, spring onions and fresh basil. Cover and cook on 100% power for 4 to 5 minutes until hot.

4. Stir in the flaked tuna and season with pepper. Cook for a further 3 minutes on 70% power until the tuna is hot. Serve garnished with basil.

NOTE: If using the microwave method, delete the Optional Kilojoules per serve.

SERVES 4

EACH SERVE PROVIDES:
4$^1/_2$ Vegetable, $^1/_4$ Fat
1$^1/_2$ Protein.
PER SERVE:
4$^1/_2$g Fat, 5$^1/_2$g Dietary Fibre.

Creamy Summer Mousse

400g peeled potatoes

1 tablespoon lemon juice

600g firm white fish fillets e.g. John Dory

3 teaspoons gelatine

¼ cup water

120g ricotta cheese

50g light sour cream

1 teaspoon horseradish sauce

Grated rind ½ lemon

1 tablespoon lemon juice

1 tablespoon chopped capers

40 mL sherry

Pepper to season

¼ cup finely sliced spring onions

¾ cup finely sliced celery

Fresh salad leaves and grated lemon rind to garnish

1. Cook the potatoes in boiling water until tender. Drain, cool and dice into 1cm cubes.

2. Sprinkle 1 tablespoon lemon juice over the fish and poach in a pan of water. Alternatively, cook in a covered microwave-safe dish on 100% power for 3 to 4 minutes. Cool and flake into small pieces. You should have 480g cooked weight.

3. Add the gelatine to the ¼ cup water and leave to swell. Dissolve over hot water or place in the microwave on 100% power for 10 seconds.

4. In a bowl, combine the ricotta, sour cream, horseradish sauce, lemon rind, lemon juice, capers, sherry and pepper. Fold in the potatoes, fish, spring onions, celery and dissolved gelatine.

5. Spoon into a 6-cup capacity ring mould. Chill until set.

6. Unmould onto a serving platter and garnish with fresh salad leaves and grated lemon rind.

Variation

▶ Substitute fresh fish fillets with 480g canned salmon or tuna, or try other seafood such as mussels or prawns.

SERVES 4

EACH SERVE PROVIDES:
½ Vegetable, 2½ Protein,
1 Bread,
150 Optional Kilojoules.
PER SERVE:
10g Fat, 3g Dietary Fibre.

Tuna on Pasta

2 cups broccoli florets

2 cups chopped fresh tomatoes

1 teaspoon garlic powder

40g sliced black olives

1 cup tomato purée

240g canned tuna in water

Pepper to season

2 tablespoons each chopped fresh parsley and celery leaves

4 cups cooked spiral pasta, hot

80g Parmesan cheese

1. Blanch the broccoli and place in a saucepan with the tomatoes, garlic powder, olives and tomato purée. Toss over a moderate heat.

2. Flake the tuna but do not drain. Add the tuna and its water to the sauce. Season with pepper and add the parsley and celery leaves.

3. Toss into the hot pasta and serve with Parmesan cheese.

Variation

▶ If you wish, you can also add two Protein serves of tuna and omit the Parmesan cheese.

Cook's Tips

▶ The broccoli florets should be small. If you do not have any broccoli, use beans or zucchini.

▶ This pasta dish is full of flavours. You can enjoy it hot when freshly made, or cold as a salad.

SERVES 4

EACH SERVE PROVIDES:
2¹/₂ Vegetable,
2 Protein, 2 Bread,
25 Optional Kilojoules.
PER SERVE:
4g Fat, 9g Dietary Fibre.

Tuna on Pasta.

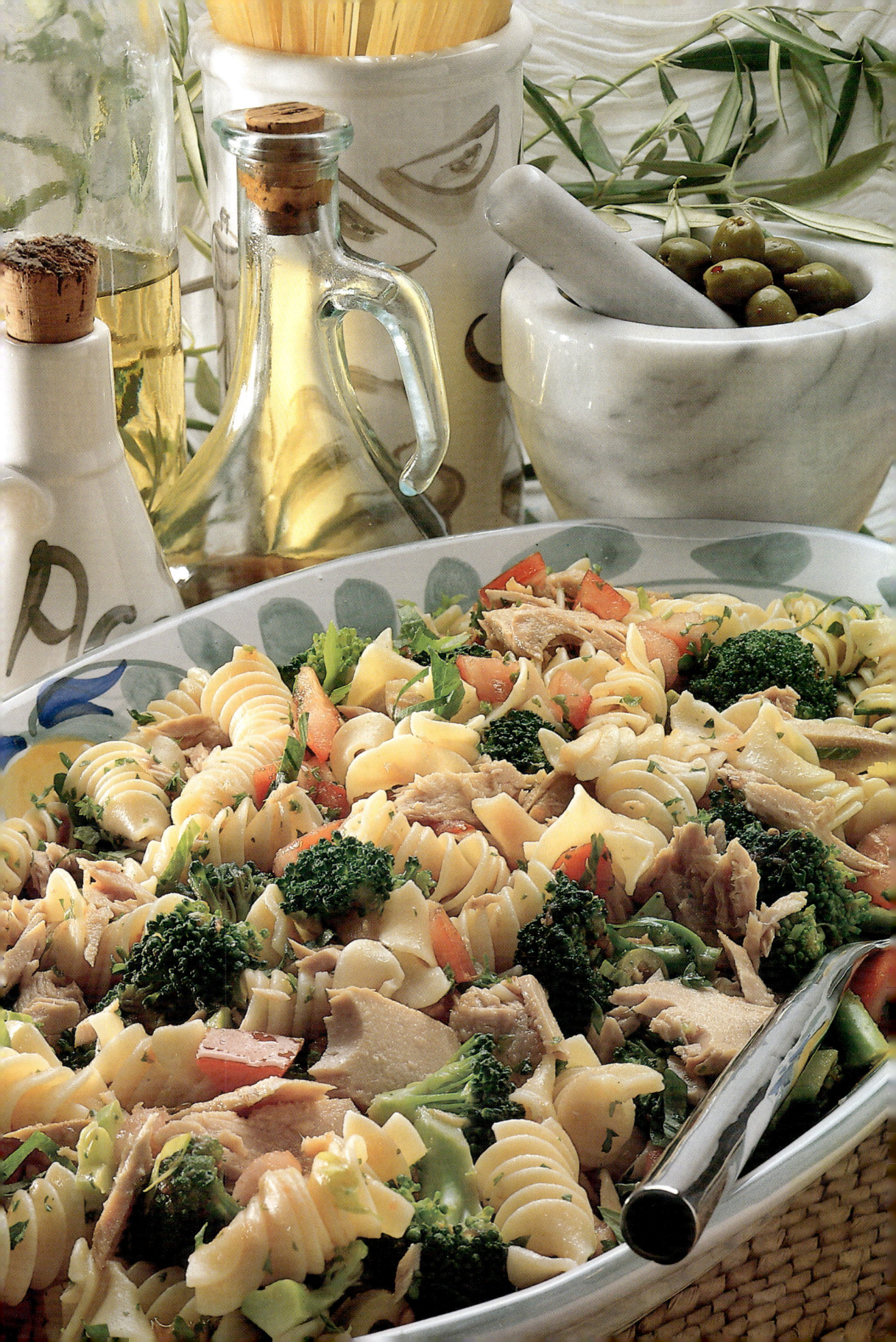

Stir-fried Squid

600g squid tubes

1 teaspoon each sesame oil and peanut oil

2 teaspoons finely chopped fresh ginger

1 green chilli, seeded and chopped

1 cup diced red capsicum

1 cup sliced bok choy stalks

3 cups chopped bok choy leaves

100g water chestnuts, halved

1/2 cup spring onions, cut into 3cm pieces

1 tablespoon oyster sauce

1 tablespoon rice wine vinegar or cider vinegar

3 1/2 cups cooked vermicelli or egg noodles, hot

1. Cut the squid tubes down one side and open out flat. Using a sharp knife, score the inside of the tubes in a criss cross pattern. Do not cut all the way through. Cut into 3cm cubes.

2. Heat the oils in a wok and add the ginger and chilli. Cook for 30 seconds over a high heat. Reduce the heat and add the capsicum and bok choy stalks, stirring continuously for 2 minutes.

3. Raise the heat and add the squid, bok choy leaves, water chestnuts and spring onions. Stir-fry for 2 to 3 minutes or until the squid tubes start to curl and whiten and the bok choy leaves wilt slightly but are still crisp.

4. Stir in the oyster sauce, vinegar and vermicelli. Serve immediately.

Cook's Tip

▶ Sesame oil adds great flavour to a lot of dishes. Do not use too much, as the flavour can be overpowering. Store in a cool, dark place.

SERVES 4

EACH SERVE PROVIDES:
3 Vegetable, 1/2 Fat,
2 Protein, 2 Bread,
20 Optional Kilojoules.
PER SERVE:
5 1/2g Fat 4g Dietary Fibre.

Scallop Salad

300g scallops

2 cups fish stock

2 cups sliced zucchini

2 cups sliced beans
(green or yellow)

1 cup asparagus spears

4 cups torn lettuce leaves

DRESSING

2 small juicy tomatoes

1 small clove garlic,
peeled

$^1/_4$ cup fresh basil leaves

4 teaspoons olive oil

2 tablespoons
white wine vinegar

Pepper to season
(optional)

1. Clean the scallops and trim any dark pieces. Heat the stock in a large frying pan to simmer. Add the scallops and poach gently for about 5 to 7 minutes until just cooked. Do not overcook as they will become tough. Drain and discard stock. Weigh to make sure you have 240g.

2. Bring a large saucepan of water to the boil and blanch the zucchini, beans and asparagus for about 3 minutes. Drain and refresh in cold water. Dry the vegetables well on absorbent paper.

3. Take the cooled scallops and slice each one into thirds to form thin, round slices.

4. In a large bowl, toss the scallops, zucchini, beans and asparagus with the lettuce leaves and dressing. Serve on four large plates.

5. To make the dressing, roast the tomatoes in the oven at 240°C for about 10 to 15 minutes until lightly browned and cooked. Blend or process with the garlic until smooth. Strain to remove the seeds and skin. Add the chopped basil leaves, olive oil and vinegar. Season with pepper if desired.

Variations

▶ If you do not have fish stock, simmer 2 cups water with 1 tablespoon vinegar, a sprig of parsley and a few peppercorns. Discard stock after cooking the scallops.

▶ Try using lettuce such as rocket, watercress, red oak, and endive (witloof). Add delicate sprouts like snow peas and then for body use butter (butterhead) lettuce.

Cook's Tips

▶ Accompany this salad with new season potatoes tossed in fresh mint.

▶ Make sure your lettuce is crisp and dry before tossing. To get the perfect lettuce leaf, wash in cold water, dry in a salad spinner or tea-towel and then wrap in a clean tea-towel and refrigerate for about 30 minutes before using. The leaves will crisp up beautifully.

SERVES 4

EACH SERVE PROVIDES:
$4^1/_2$ Vegetable, 1 Fat,
1 Protein.
PER SERVE:
6g Fat, 5g Dietary Fibre.

Prawn Risotto

4 teaspoons olive oil

1 cup chopped onion

2 cloves garlic, crushed

160g arborio rice

2¾ cups fish stock

300g shelled and
deveined green prawns

2 cups very finely
shredded cabbage

80g grated
Parmesan cheese

½ teaspoon black pepper

Chopped Italian parsley
to garnish

1 Heat the olive oil in a large saucepan and add the onion and garlic. Cook over a low heat for about 15 minutes until the onion is soft but not coloured.

2 Mix in the rice.

3 Add ½ cup fish stock and stir constantly until the rice has absorbed all the liquid. Gradually add the remaining stock, ½ cup at a time, until all the stock has been added and the rice is tender. Do not rush the process or the rice will catch to the saucepan.

4 Cut the prawns in halves or thirds, depending on their size. When the rice is just cooked, stir through the prawns and cabbage. Cover and cook for a few minutes only, until the prawns have turned pink, the cabbage is slightly wilted and the rice tender.

5 Add the Parmesan cheese and pepper. Serve in bowls, garnished with Italian parsley.

Variation

▶ If you cannot buy green (raw) prawns, use 240g shelled and deveined cooked prawns. Add them halfway through cooking the cabbage, just long enough to warm through.

Cook's Tip

▶ Fish stock should be quite mild in flavour. The packet stocks can be strong. As fish bones have no fat, you can make your own. Ask for fish ribs, preferably from snapper, Dory or similar. Cover the bones with water, a chopped onion, a celery stalk and few peppercorns. Simmer for 20 minutes only, then strain.

SERVES 4

EACH SERVE PROVIDES:
1½ Vegetable, 1 Fat,
2 Protein, 2 Bread,
35 Optional Kilojoules.
PER SERVE:
13g Fat, 2½g Dietary Fibre.

Prawn Risotto (bottom); Spicy Mussels with Noodles (page 30).

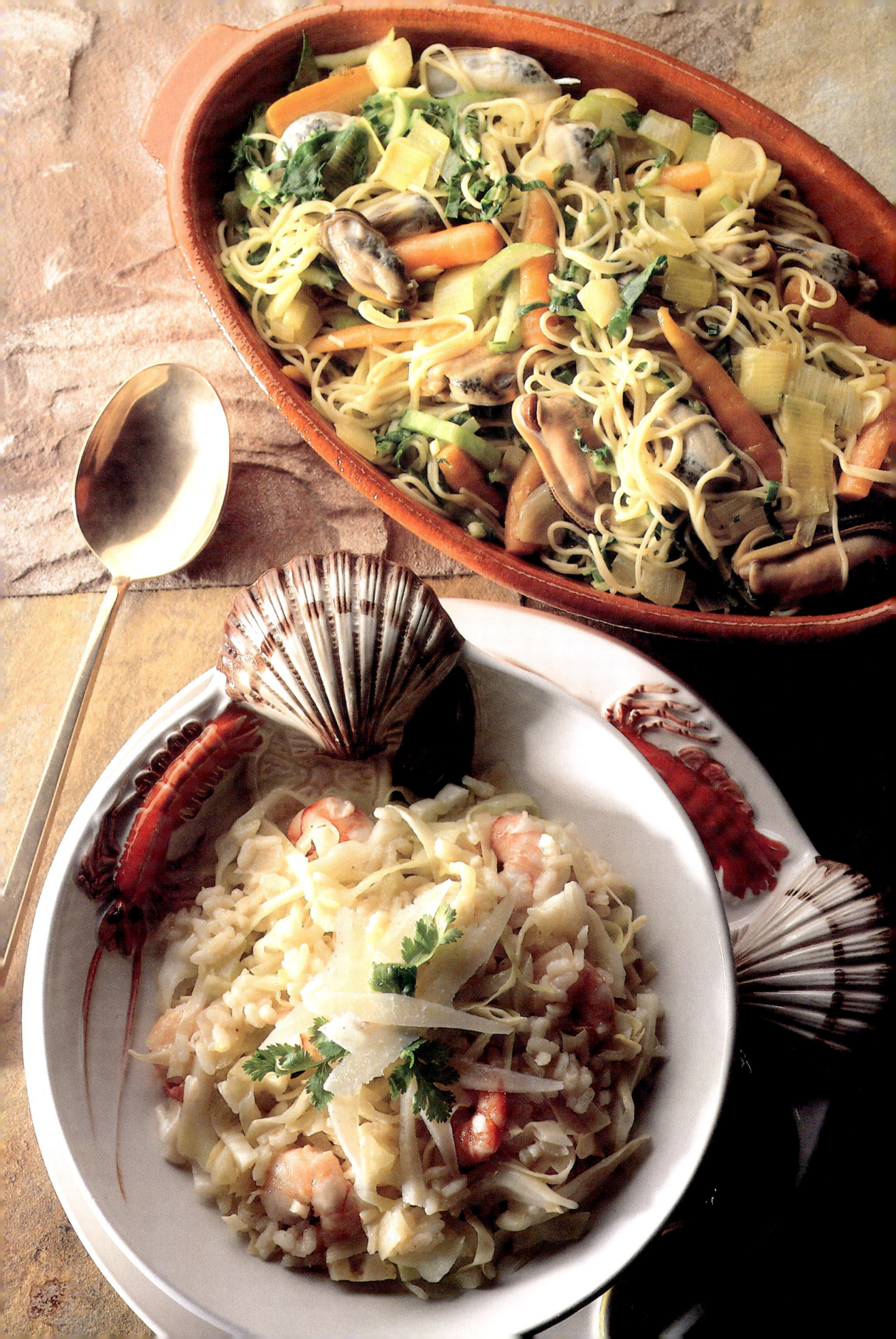

Spicy Mussels with Noodles

240g cooked mussels

4 teaspoons vegetable oil

1 clove garlic, crushed

$^1/_2$ cup chopped onion

$^1/_2$ cup chopped leeks

2 cups sliced baby carrots

1 teaspoon
mild curry powder

$1^1/_2$ cups vegetable stock

1 tablespoon cornflour

1 teaspoon
prepared mild mustard

2 cups sliced bok choy

25g light cream cheese

4 cups cooked
egg noodles, hot

1. Cut the mussels in half if they are large.

2. Heat the oil in a frying pan and cook the garlic, onion, leeks, carrots and curry powder over a moderate heat for about 5 minutes.

3. Blend the vegetable stock, cornflour and mustard, and stir into the pan.

4. Add the mussels, bok choy and cream cheese. Bring to the boil and simmer for 2 to 3 minutes until heated through. Toss through freshly cooked noodles.

Cook's Tip

▶ If you have some fresh oregano or basil, add 2 or 3 table-spoons of chopped fresh herbs to this recipe. It will add to the flavour.

SERVES 4

EACH SERVE PROVIDES:
$2^1/_2$ Vegetable, 1 Fat,
1 Protein, 2 Bread,
120 Optional Kilojoules.
PER SERVE:
9g Fat, 7g Dietary Fibre.

Pictured page 29.

Tuna Bake

2 cups skim milk

2 tablespoons cornflour

4 cups cauliflower florets

360g canned tuna in water, drained and flaked

$^1/_2$ cup chopped spring onions

$^1/_2$ cup gherkins, chopped

2 hard-cooked eggs, chopped

$1^1/_2$ tablespoons chopped fresh dill

Pepper to season (optional)

1 slice wholemeal bread, crumbed

40g grated fresh Parmesan cheese

1. Heat $1^1/_2$ cups milk in a saucepan. Mix the cornflour with the extra milk and stir in. Cook, stirring until the sauce thickens. Remove from the heat and set aside.

2. Blanch the cauliflower and add to the sauce with the tuna, spring onions, gherkins, eggs and dill. Season with pepper if desired.

3. Turn into a casserole dish. Sprinkle over the breadcrumbs and Parmesan. Bake at 180°C for 30 minutes until hot and golden brown.

Microwave Method

1. Heat $1^1/_2$ cups milk in the microwave until it reaches boiling point, about $2^1/_2$ minutes on 100% power.

2. Blend the cornflour with the remaining milk and combine with the hot milk. Cook on 100% for a further 3 minutes until the sauce thickens, stirring occasionally. Set aside.

3. In a separate microwave-safe bowl, add the cauliflower with a dash of water. Cover and cook on 100% power for 4 minutes until just cooked. Drain well.

4. Add the cooked cauliflower to the sauce with the tuna, spring onions, gherkins, eggs and dill. Season with pepper if desired.

5. Turn the mixture into a microwave-safe casserole dish. Cover and cook on 70% power for 4 minutes until hot.

6. Sprinkle over the breadcrumbs and grated Parmesan. Place under the grill for about 3 to 4 minutes until golden.

Cook's Tip

▶ Serve with seasonal vegetables.

SERVES 4

EACH SERVE PROVIDES:
$2^1/_2$ Vegetable, $2^1/_2$ Protein,
$^1/_4$ Bread, $^1/_2$ Milk,
100 Optional Kilojoules.
PER SERVE:
$9^1/_2$g Fat, $3^1/_2$g Dietary Fibre.

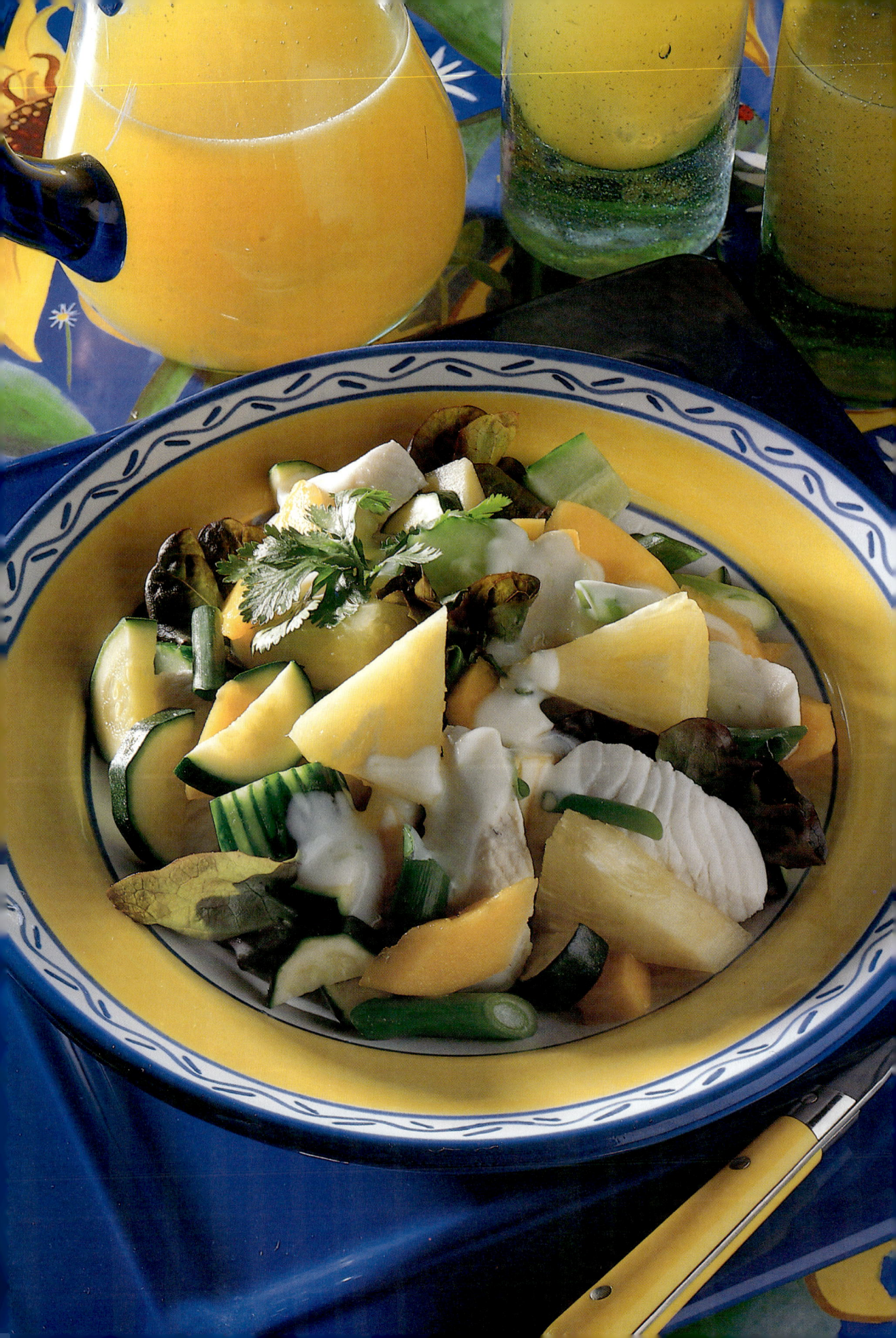

Tropical Seafood Salad

600g firm white fish fillets e.g John Dory

$^1/_4$ cup lime juice

1 teaspoon chopped fresh chilli

$^1/_2$ cup chopped spring onions

2 cups chopped pawpaw

1 cup chopped pineapple pieces

$1^1/_2$ cups peeled chopped cucumber

1 cup snow peas or sliced zucchini, blanched and trimmed

Grated lime or lemon rind to garnish

DRESSING

$^3/_4$ cup natural low-fat yoghurt

Few drops coconut essence

$1^1/_2$ tablespoons chopped fresh coriander

1 teaspoon grated lime or lemon rind

1. Cut the fish fillets into 2cm pieces. Toss with the lime juice and chilli. Marinate for 1 hour in the refrigerator.

2. Poach or grill the fish until just tender. Alternatively, place in a microwave-safe dish, cover and cook on 100% power for $3^1/_2$ to 4 minutes until just cooked. You should have 480g cooked weight.

3. In a separate bowl, mix the spring onions, pawpaw, pineapple, cucumber and snow peas with the combined dressing ingredients.

4. Gently fold in the fish. Pile equal amounts of fish onto lettuce filled bowls. Garnish with lime rind to serve.

Cook's Tip

▶ Serve with oven baked sweet potatoes and yoghurt, or try pappadums cooked in the microwave.

SERVES 4

EACH SERVE PROVIDES:
1 Fruit, $1^1/_2$ Vegetable,
2 Protein,
140 Optional Kilojoules.
PER SERVE:
$4^1/_2$g Fat, $4^1/_2$g Dietary Fibre.

Tropical Seafood Salad.

Thai Grilled Fish

4x150g firm white fish fillets e.g. John Dory

Fresh basil and mint to garnish

MARINADE

2 stalks lemon grass

1 clove garlic, crushed

1 teaspoon chopped fresh ginger

2 tablespoons chopped fresh coriander

$\frac{1}{2}$ teaspoon chilli paste

Juice 1 lime or $\frac{1}{2}$ lemon

1. To prepare the marinade, trim the lemon grass stalks, discarding any green part. You need only keep the tender white parts.

2. Blend or process the lemon grass, garlic, ginger, coriander, chilli paste and lime juice, until smooth.

3. To prepare the fish, cut each fillet into finger width pieces. Toss the fish in the marinade. Cover and refrigerate for 1 hour.

4. Heat the grill until very hot. Arrange the fish in one layer on a foil-lined baking tray. Grill for 3 to 4 minutes, turning once or twice until the fish is cooked. Garnish with basil and mint.

Microwave Method

While grilling will give the fish a lovely colour and is the preferred cooking method for this recipe, you can also microwave the fish.

1. Follow the recipe steps 1, 2 and 3.

2. Arrange the fish in one layer on a microwave-safe dish. Cover with plastic wrap and cook on 70% power for $3\frac{1}{2}$ to 4 minutes. Leave for 1 minute before serving. Garnish with basil and mint.

Cook's Tips

▶ Serve on a bed of rice with one serve of pawpaw and fresh salad greens. Yoghurt and cucumber slices make a nice accompaniment to this dish. Mix $\frac{1}{2}$ cup grated cucumber with $\frac{1}{2}$ cup natural low-fat yoghurt. Toss in 1 tablespoon chopped fresh mint.

▶ If you prefer toss the cooked fish through mixed salad greens with yoghurt and serve as a warm salad.

SERVES 4

EACH SERVE PROVIDES:
2 Protein.
PER SERVE:
4g Fat, $\frac{1}{2}$g Dietary Fibre.

Thai Grilled Fish served with lettuce greens, rice and pawpaw.

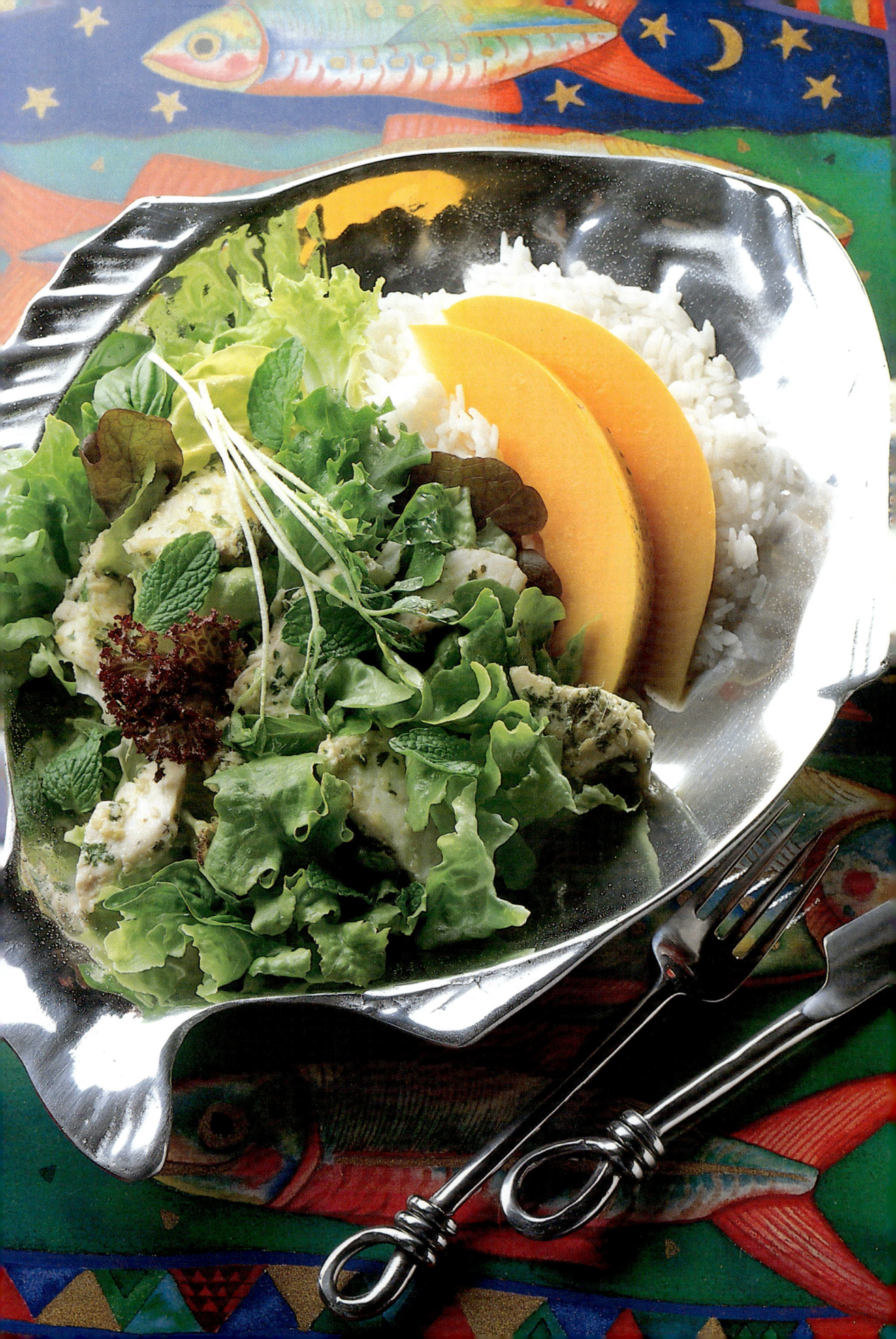

Lemon and Ginger Fillets

600g firm white fish fillets e.g. John Dory

Chopped fresh coriander and 1 teaspoon finely grated lemon rind to garnish

SAUCE

$^1/_2$ teaspoon sesame oil

2 teaspoons finely chopped fresh ginger

1 cup sliced celery, cut diagonally

Grated rind and juice 1 lemon

2 teaspoons honey

$^3/_4$ cup chicken stock

3 teaspoons cornflour

$^1/_2$ cup chopped spring onions

$1^1/_2$ cups drained sliced baby corn

100g drained water chestnuts

1 cup mung bean sprouts

1. To prepare the sauce, heat the oil in a pan and cook the ginger and celery over a moderate heat for 1 to 2 minutes.

2. Add the lemon rind, juice, honey, stock and cornflour, heating only until thickened. Stir in the spring onions, baby corn, water chestnuts and sprouts, and heat through.

3. Grill the fish on a foil-lined baking tray.

4. Arrange the fish on plates, spoon over the sauce and garnish with the coriander and lemon rind.

Microwave Method

1. To prepare the sauce, put the oil, ginger and celery in a microwave-safe bowl, cover and cook on 100% power for 2 minutes.

2. In a jug, mix the lemon rind and juice, honey, chicken stock and cornflour. Pour into the celery mixture and stir well. Cover and cook on 100% power for a further 3 minutes until thickened.

3. Stir in the spring onions, baby corn, water chestnuts and bean sprouts.

4. Tuck the thinner ends of the fish underneath so the fish is the same thickness throughout. Place in a microwave-safe dish, cover and cook on 100% power for $3^1/_2$ to 4 minutes or until the fish is just cooked. Leave for 1 minute.

5. Arrange the fish on plates. Reheat the sauce and spoon over the fish. Garnish with coriander and lemon rind.

Cook's Tips

▶ If you do not fold the thinner ends of each fish fillet underneath when microwave cooking, you will find that these ends will overcook and toughen.

▶ Accompany with steamed jasmine rice which has been cooked with a strip of lemon peel in the water.

SERVES 4

EACH SERVE PROVIDES:
$1^1/_4$ Vegetable,
2 Protein, 1 Bread,
120 Optional Kilojoules.
PER SERVE:
5g Fat, 6g Dietary Fibre.

Parmesan Crumbed Fish

4x150g firm white fish fillets e.g. John Dory

Lemon juice to serve

2 tablespoons chopped fresh parsley to garnish

TOPPING

40g grated Parmesan cheese

2 slices wholemeal bread, crumbed

1 tablespoon chopped capers

Juice of 1 lemon

2 teaspoons olive oil

Pepper to season

1. To prepare the topping, in a bowl mix the Parmesan, breadcrumbs, capers, lemon juice and olive oil. Season with pepper.

2. Spread the topping evenly over the four fillets. Place them on a foil-lined baking tray and grill under a moderate heat for about 5 minutes until the fish is cooked. Do not have the temperature too high, as the topping will burn before the fish is cooked.

3. Squeeze over the lemon juice and serve garnished with chopped parsley.

Microwave Method

1. Combine the topping ingredients in a bowl.

2. Arrange the fish in one layer in a microwave-safe dish, tucking the thinner ends underneath so the fish is the same thickness throughout.

3. Spread the topping evenly over the four fillets.

4. Cover with plastic wrap and cook on 70% power for about 4 to 5 minutes (depending on the thickness of the fillets). Leave for 1 minute.

5. Squeeze over the lemon juice and garnish with parsley.

Cook's Tip

▶ If you microwave this dish, you get a soft topping but if you grill the fish, you get a crisp coating. Whichever way you choose, it will taste delicious.

SERVES 4

EACH SERVE PROVIDES:
$^1/_2$ Fat, $2^1/_2$ Protein,
$^1/_2$ Bread.
PER SERVE:
10g Fat, 1g Dietary Fibre.

Salmon Couscous

4x150g boneless salmon
fillets

1–2 tablespoons lemon
juice

Fresh dill and lemon
slices to garnish

SALAD

160g couscous

1¼ cups boiling
vegetable stock

4 large juicy tomatoes

2 cups finely sliced celery

2 tablespoons chopped
fresh dill

4 teaspoons olive oil

¼ cup white wine or
tarragon vinegar

Pepper to season

1. To prepare the salad, put the couscous in a large bowl and pour over the boiling stock. Cover and set aside for 5 minutes until the couscous has absorbed all the stock.

2. Blanch and peel the tomatoes. Cut them in half lengthways, squeeze out the seeds and discard. Cut the tomato flesh into thin strips. You should have 2 cups.

3. Mix the couscous, tomatoes, celery, dill, olive oil, vinegar and pepper, tossing gently with your hands.

4. Place the salmon fillets in a microwave-safe dish and sprinkle with lemon juice. Cover loosely with plastic and cook on 100% power for 4 minutes or until the salmon is almost cooked. Leave for about 1 minute. Alternatively, heat 1 cup of water in a frying pan and poach the salmon gently for 2 to 3 minutes each side. Set aside and discard the cooking water.

5. Divide the couscous salad equally between four serving bowls. Top each with a salmon fillet. Serve garnished with extra dill and lemon slices.

Variation

▶ In place of couscous, use 4 cups cooked burghul wheat or cooked rice. Brown rice or gourmet blends of rice would be delicious.

SERVES 4

EACH SERVE PROVIDES:
3 Vegetable, 1 Fat,
2 Protein, 2 Bread,
15 Optional Kilojoules.
PER SERVE:
10g Fat, 7g Dietary Fibre.

Salmon Couscous.

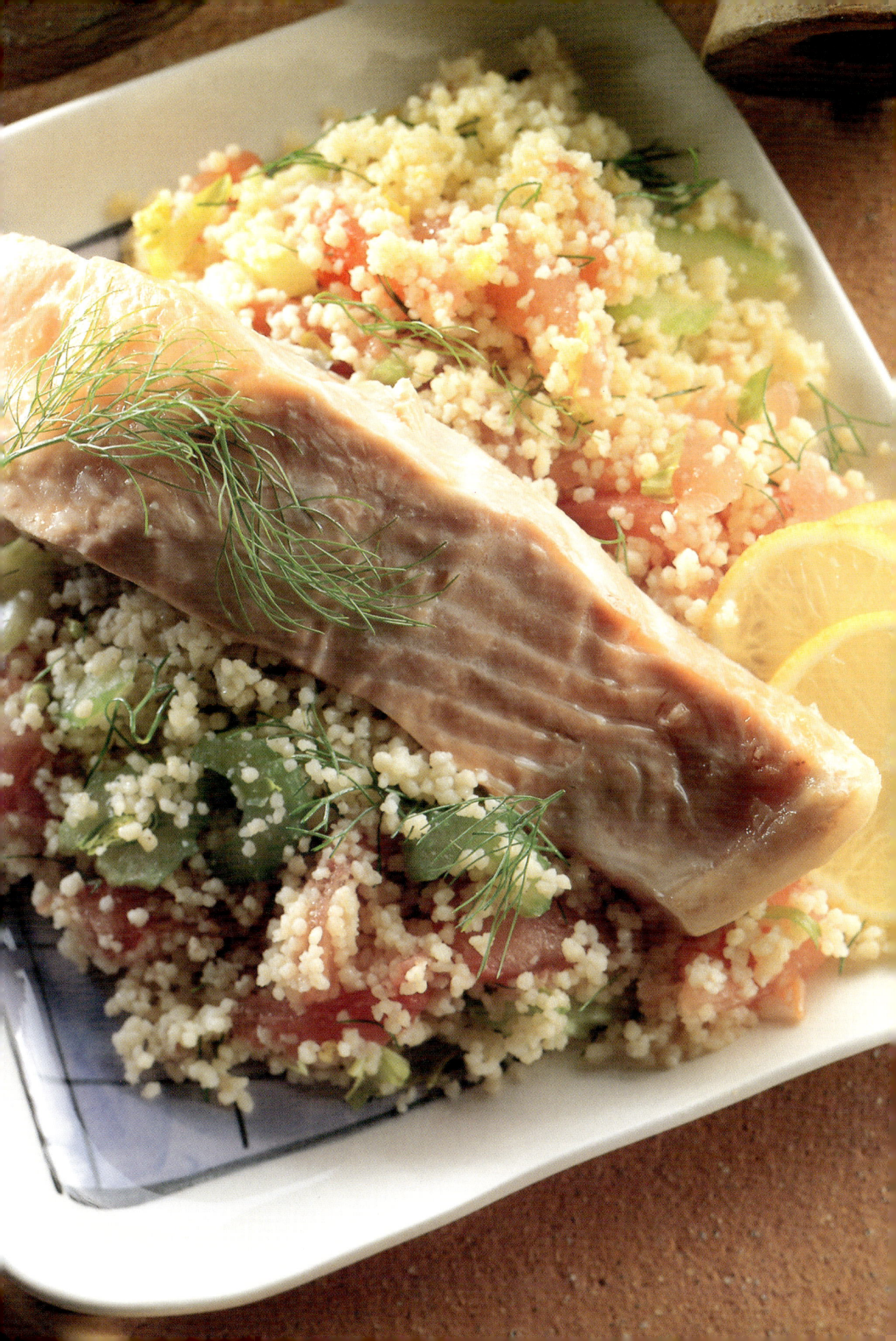

Five Spiced Salmon

½ cup sliced spring onions

1 tablespoon chopped fresh ginger

2 teaspoons olive oil

½ teaspoon five spice powder

Good shake garlic salt

4x150g salmon fillets or steaks

¼ cup fish stock

1. In a bowl, mix the spring onions, ginger, oil, five spice powder and garlic salt.

2. Spread the mixture evenly over the salmon fillets.

3. Grill under a moderate heat for 5 to 6 minutes until the salmon is cooked. Brush with the fish stock while grilling to moisten.

Microwave Method

1. Mix the spring onions, ginger, oil, five spice powder and garlic salt in a small microwave-safe bowl and cover with plastic wrap. Cook on 100% power for 1 minute.

2. Arrange the salmon fillets in a circle in a microwave-safe dish. If you are using steaks, put the thicker end of each steak towards the outside edge of the dish.

3. Spread the spring onion mixture evenly over the top of the salmon. Pour over the stock and cover with plastic wrap.

4. Cook on 70% power for 4 minutes. Leave for 1 minute. Serve hot or chilled.

Variation

▶ Rather than using all olive oil, you can use half olive oil and a dash of sesame oil for a more interesting flavour. Try these salmon steaks on the barbecue as well.

SERVES 4

EACH SERVE PROVIDES:
¼ Vegetable, ½ Fat,
2 Protein,
5 Optional Kilojoules.
PER SERVE:
6½g Fat, ½g Dietary Fibre.

Mushroom Topped Fillets

4x150g firm white fish fillets e.g. John Dory

1 tablespoon lemon juice

Pepper to season

SAUCE

4 teaspoons vegetable oil

2¹/₂ cups sliced mushrooms

¹/₂ cup sliced spring onions

1 tablespoon chopped fresh dill or 1 teaspoon dried

1 teaspoon paprika

60mL dry sherry

¹/₄ cup water

2 teaspoons cornflour

50g light sour cream

1. To prepare the sauce, heat the oil in a frying pan and cook the mushrooms for 2 to 3 minutes. Add the spring onions, dill, paprika and sherry. Simmer for 2 to 3 minutes.

2. Blend the water and cornflour, add the sour cream, and stir in. Cook until the sauce thickens.

3. Drizzle the lemon juice over the the fish fillets and grill until cooked. Season with pepper and serve with the sauce.

Microwave Method

1. Cook the sliced mushrooms, spring onions, dill, paprika and sherry in a microwave-safe dish on 100% power for 3 minutes.

2. Drizzle the lemon juice over the fillets and arrange in a single layer in a microwave-safe dish. Tuck the thinner ends of the fish underneath so the fish is the same thickness throughout.

3. Mix the water and cornflour, stir into the mushroom mixture, add the sour cream and pour over the fish.

4. Cover with plastic wrap and cook on 70% power for 4 minutes. Stand for 1 minute. Season with pepper and serve.

NOTE: If using the microwave method, delete 1 Fat Selection per serve.

Cook's Tip

▶ Serve with seasonal vegetables and rice or potatoes.

SERVES 4

EACH SERVE PROVIDES:
1¹/₂ Vegetable, 1 Fat,
2 Protein,
225 Optional Kilojoules.
PER SERVE:
12g Fat, 1¹/₂g Dietary Fibre.

Fish with Grapes and Ginger

4 x 150g firm white fish
fillets e.g. John Dory

1 tablespoon lemon juice

4 cups cooked rice, hot

Chopped fresh coriander
and sliced ginger
to garnish

SAUCE

4 teaspoons olive oil

1 cup finely diced onion

2 teaspoons finely
chopped fresh ginger

$\frac{1}{2}$ teaspoon cumin

$1\frac{1}{2}$ teaspoons ground
coriander

$\frac{3}{4}$ cup vegetable or
fish stock

15mL sherry

1 tablespoon cornflour

$\frac{1}{4}$ cup natural
low-fat yoghurt

100g green grapes,
preferably seedless

1. To prepare the sauce, heat the oil in a frying pan. Add the onion and ginger, and cook for 2 to 3 minutes. Stir in the cumin and coriander, and cook for several minutes.

2. Mix the stock with the sherry and cornflour. Stir into the sauce and simmer until the sauce thickens. Add the yoghurt and grapes, stirring until heated. Do not allow the sauce to boil.

3. Sprinkle the fish fillets with lemon juice and poach or grill until tender.

4. To serve, place equal quantities of rice on each plate. Top with a fillet of fish and spoon over the sauce. Garnish with coriander and ginger.

Microwave Method

1. To prepare the sauce, put the onion and ginger into a microwave-safe bowl with a splash of water and cover loosely. Cook on 100% power for 4 minutes.

2. Stir in the cumin and coriander, and cook for a further 1 minute on 100% power.

3. Combine the stock, sherry, cornflour and yoghurt and stir in. Cook on 100% power for $1\frac{1}{2}$ to 2 minutes until the sauce thickens. Fold in the grapes.

4. In another flat microwave dish, arrange the fish fillets. Tuck the thinner ends underneath so the fish is the same thickness throughout.

5. Sprinkle the fish with the lemon juice. Cover loosely and cook on 100% power for $3\frac{1}{2}$ to 4 minutes or until just cooked, depending on the thickness of the fillets. Leave for 1 minute.

6. Serve with rice, garnished with coriander and ginger. See Step 4 above.

NOTE: If using the microwave method, delete 1 Fat Selection per serve.

SERVES 4

EACH SERVE PROVIDES:
$\frac{1}{4}$ Fruit, $\frac{1}{2}$ Vegetable,
1 Fat, 2 Protein, 2 Bread,
115 Optional Kilojoules.
PER SERVE:
$9\frac{1}{2}$g Fat, $2\frac{1}{2}$g Dietary Fibre.

Fish with Grapes and Ginger.

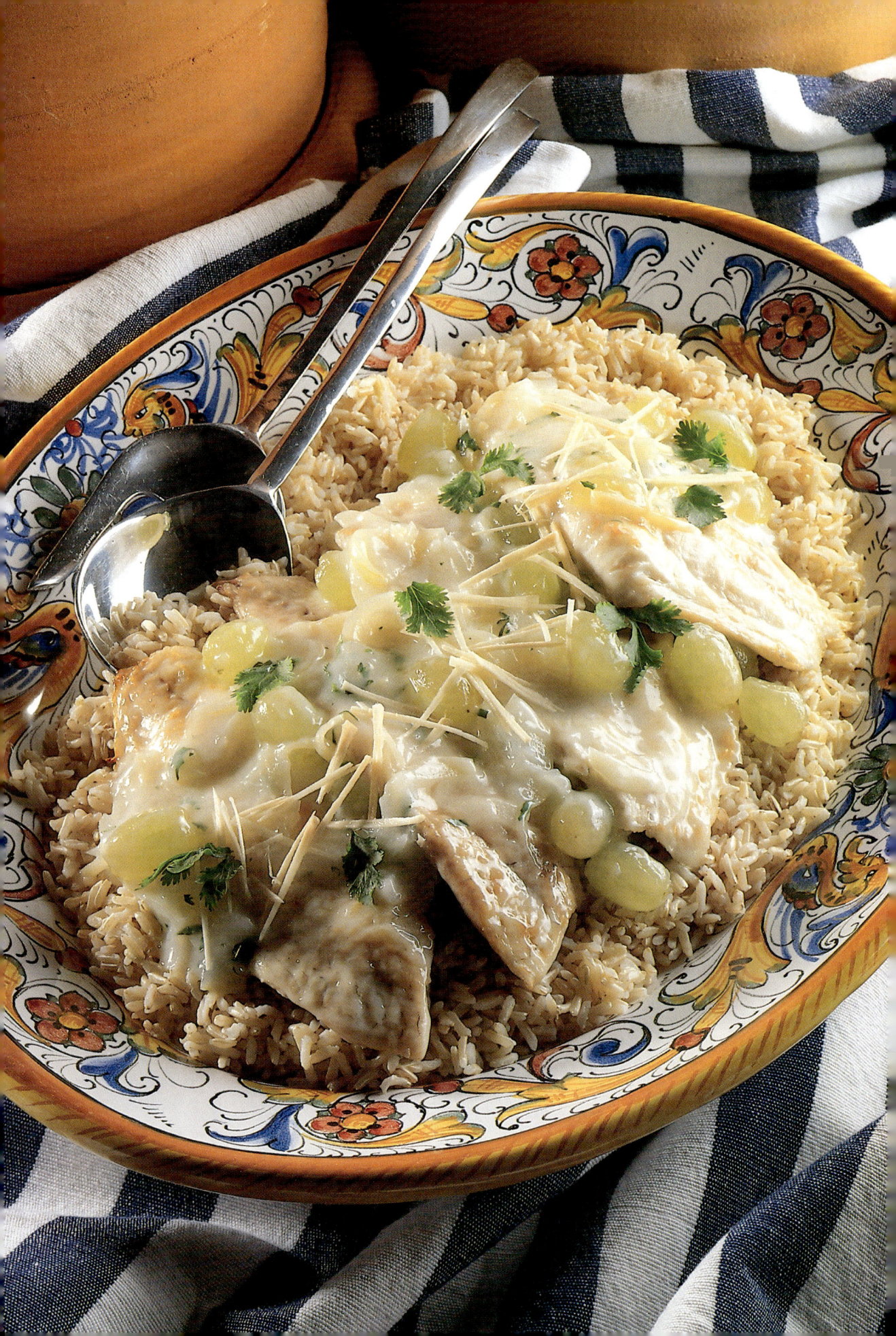

Baked Fish with Capsicum

600g firm white fish fillets e.g. John Dory, no skin

3½ cups cooked spaghetti, hot

Fresh basil to garnish

SAUCE

1 cup finely chopped onion

1 cup chopped yellow capsicum

1 tablespoon tomato paste

1½ cups chopped canned tomatoes

1 tablespoon chopped fresh basil

Pepper to season

STUFFING

6 sun-dried tomato halves (not packed in oil)

1 tablespoon chopped fresh basil

1½ slices wholemeal bread, crumbed

20g grated Parmesan cheese

20g stuffed olives, chopped

Microwave Method

1 To prepare the sauce, put the onion and capsicum in a microwave-safe bowl with a splash of water, cover and cook on 100% power for 4 minutes. Set aside 2 table-spoons for the stuffing. Add the tomato paste and cook for 2 minutes. Mix in the chopped tomatoes and fresh basil, and season with pepper.

2 To prepare the stuffing, pour ¼ cup boiling water over the sun-dried tomato halves and leave for 5 minutes. Drain, reserving the water, and slice the tomatoes.

3 In a bowl, combine the dried tomatoes, basil, breadcrumbs, Parmesan, olives, 2 tablespoons reserved capsicum mixture and about 2 tablespoons of reserved sun-dried tomato water to moisten the stuffing.

4 Place the fish on a board and spread equal quantities of stuffing over each fillet. Roll up the fillets and secure with a toothpick.

5 Stand the fillets upright in a microwave-safe serving dish. Spoon over the sauce.

6 Cover loosely and cook on 100% power for 5 to 6 minutes until the sauce is hot and the fish tender. Serve with hot spaghetti, garnished with fresh basil.

SERVES 4

EACH SERVE PROVIDES:
2½ Vegetable, 2¼ Protein,
2 Bread,
55 Optional Kilojoules.
PER SERVE:
7g Fat, 6½g Dietary Fibre.

Chunky Fish Casserole

1¹/₂ cups sliced leeks

2 cups diced pumpkin

1 cup skim milk

600g firm white fish fillets e.g. John Dory

1¹/₂ cups diced zucchini

¹/₂ teaspoon paprika

1 cup creamed corn

1¹/₂ tablespoons Italian flat parsley

40g Parmesan cheese

Ground black pepper to season

4x60g bread rolls

Microwave Method

1. Put the leeks, pumpkin and milk into a large microwave-safe casserole dish. Cover loosely and cook on 100% power for 6 to 7 minutes until the pumpkin is tender.

2. Dice the fish in large pieces and add to the casserole with the zucchini. Cover and cook on 100% power for a further 5 minutes.

3. Add the paprika, corn, parsley and Parmesan. Season well with pepper.

4. Cook on 70% power for 4 minutes. Leave for 2 minutes and serve with warm bread rolls.

Variation

▶ Try this recipe with other seafood such as mussels, prawns and scallops. Chicken is also suitable.

SERVES 4

EACH SERVE PROVIDES:
2¹/₂ Vegetable,
2¹/₂ Protein, 2¹/₂ Bread,
¹/₄ Milk.
PER SERVE:
10g Fat, 7¹/₂g Dietary Fibre.

MAIN COURSE MEATS

At its best, meat is succulent and delicious, adding great interest to our meals. Always look for lean cuts with the fat well trimmed. Quite often, cheaper meats have more fat on them. Choose a good quality product that will give you the best taste. In addition to lamb, beef, ham and pork, we now have a wide range of chicken cuts, especially versatile and useful for quick dinners. Meat is a source of protein and iron so be sure to include it in your eating plan.

Chicken Jalouise

6 sun-dried tomato halves (not packed in oil)

¼ cup boiling water

360g boneless chicken pieces, no skin or fat

2 teaspoons olive oil

½ cup finely chopped onion

1 cup sliced celery

1 cup diced red capsicum

1 cup sliced mushrooms

1½ tablespoons tomato paste

2 teaspoons capers

1 tablespoon chopped fresh oregano

240g filo pastry

2 tablespoons skim milk

1. Put the sun-dried tomatoes and boiling water in a bowl and leave to swell while preparing the other ingredients.

2. Grill the chicken under a moderate heat for about 10 minutes until golden and tender. Turn once. Cool a little and cut into small pieces.

3. Heat the oil in a frying pan and cook the onion, celery, capsicum and mushrooms for 5 minutes. Add the tomato paste and cook for 5 minutes until the paste darkens a little.

4. Drain the sun-dried tomatoes, reserving the liquid, and slice. Add the tomatoes and liquid to the pan with the chicken, capers and oregano. Mix well and set aside.

5. Spray a baking tray with non-stick spray. Place one sheet of filo pastry on top and brush with the milk. Repeat with half the sheets. Spread the chicken filling to within 2cm of the edge of the pastry.

6. Spread the remaining sheets of filo pastry with milk and layer on top of each other. Using a sharp knife, make long cuts across the pastry, about 2cm apart and about 2cm from the edges all the way around.

7. Place on top of the chicken and press the edges together. Brush the top with a little of the remaining milk.

8. Bake at 190°C for 15 to 20 minutes or until golden and crispy. Serve immediately.

SERVES 4

EACH SERVE PROVIDES:
2½ Vegetable, ½ Fat,
2 Protein, 2 Bread,
90 Optional Kilojoules.
PER SERVE:
6g Fat, 4g Dietary Fibre.

Cook's Tip

▶ Cooking tomato paste enhances its colour and flavour. It will improve the dish whenever you use the technique.

Chicken Jalouise.

46

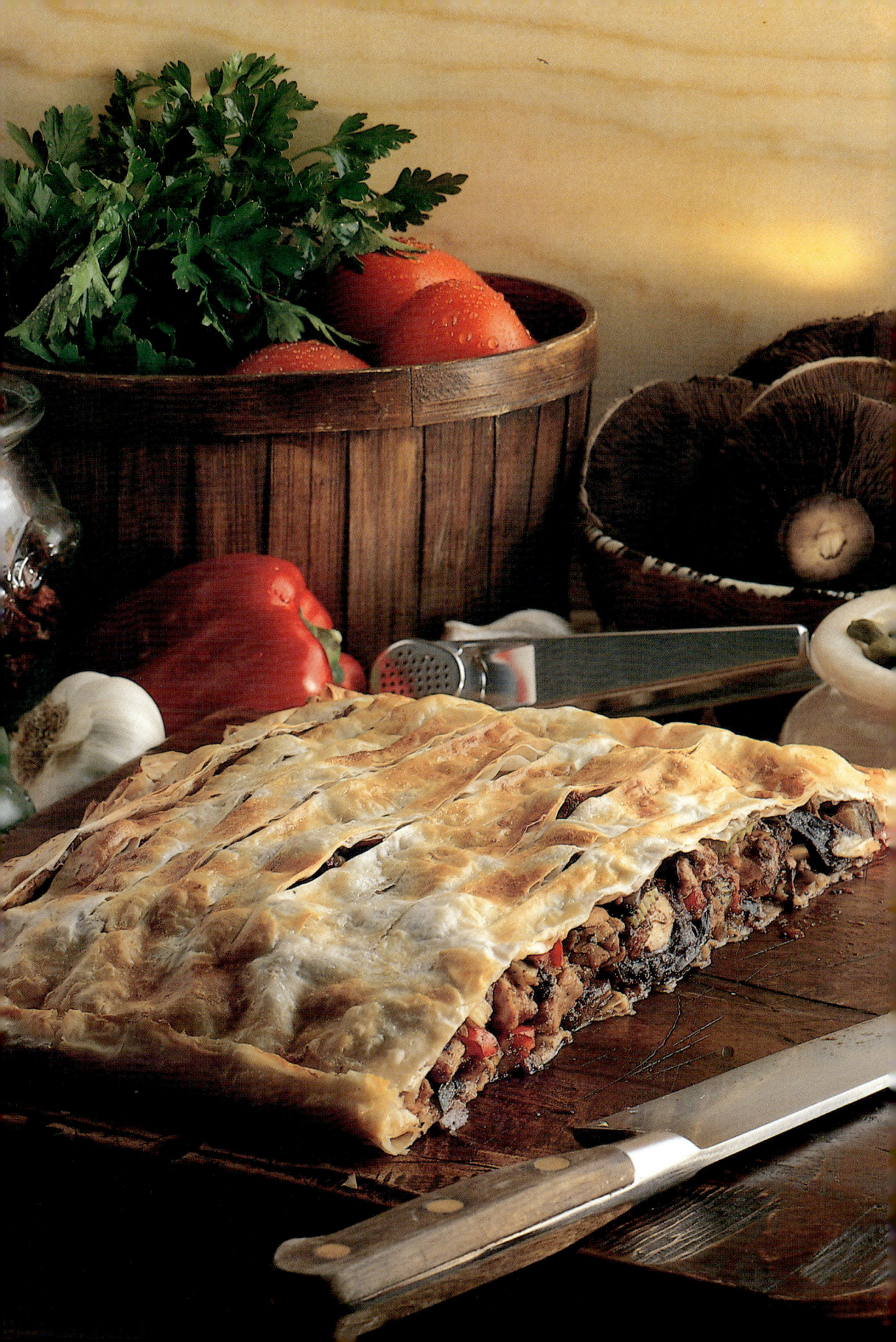

Chicken and Ham Pie

320g boneless chicken thigh pieces, no skin or fat

2 cups chicken stock

$^1/_2$ onion

1 bay leaf

Few stalks fresh parsley

Few peppercorns

$1^1/_2$ cups sliced leeks

1 cup sliced carrot

$^1/_2$ cup diced onion

60g shredded ham

$^3/_4$ cup skim milk

2 tablespoons plain flour

PASTRY TOPPING

120g filo pastry

2 tablespoons skim milk

1 In a saucepan, simmer the chicken, stock, onion, bay leaf, parsley and peppercorns for about 30 minutes until the chicken is tender. Remove the chicken from the stock and leave to cool. You should have 240g in weight.

2 Strain the stock and return to the saucepan.

3 Add the leeks, carrot, onion and ham, and simmer for about 5 minutes.

4 Mix the milk and flour, and add to the saucepan with the chicken. Cook for 3 to 5 minutes to thicken. Transfer to a casserole dish.

5 To prepare the pastry topping, brush one sheet of filo pastry with a little milk, carefully scrunch up the filo like a piece of paper and place it on top of the pie. Repeat with the remaining filo and milk.

6 Bake at 180°C for 20 minutes until the filo is well cooked and the pie is hot.

Cook's Tip

▶ Serve with seasonal vegetables.

SERVES 4

EACH SERVE PROVIDES:
$1^1/_2$ Vegetable, $2^1/_2$ Protein,
1 Bread, $^1/_4$ Milk,
125 Optional Kilojoules.
PER SERVE:
$3^1/_2$g Fat, $3^1/_2$g Dietary Fibre.

Chicken Cannelloni

140g cannelloni tubes

Chopped fresh basil
to garnish

SAUCE

1 large red capsicum

$1^1/_2$ cups canned
tomatoes in juice

FILLING

1 slice wholemeal bread,
crumbed

$^1/_2$ cup skim milk

320g minced chicken

$^1/_2$ cup grated zucchini

Grated rind
1 lemon or lime

$^1/_2$ teaspoon
white pepper

$^1/_4$ cup chopped fresh
chervil or parsley

SERVES 4

EACH SERVE PROVIDES:
$1^1/_2$ Vegetable, 2 Protein,
2 Bread,
45 Optional Kilojoules.
PER SERVE:
3g Fat, 5g Dietary Fibre.

1. To prepare the sauce, heat the grill to its maximum temperature. Grill the capsicum until it blackens and blisters. Cool in a freezer bag. Peel the charred skin from the capsicum and remove the core and seeds.

2. Blend or process the capsicum and tomatoes to make a smooth sauce. Set aside.

3. To prepare the filling, in a bowl mix the breadcrumbs with milk. Leave for 10 minutes.

4. Blend in the minced chicken, zucchini, lemon rind, pepper and chervil. Fill the cannelloni tubes with the mixture.

5. Pour half the sauce into an ovenproof dish and add the cannelloni tubes. Top with remaining sauce. Bake at 180°C for 40 to 45 minutes until hot and the tubes are cooked. Serve garnished with basil.

Microwave Method

1. Follow the recipe steps 1, 2, 3 and 4.

2. Pour half the sauce into a microwave-safe dish and place the cannelloni tubes on top. Pour over the remaining sauce.

3. Cook on 70% power for 10 minutes. Leave for 4 minutes. Serve garnished with basil.

Variation

▶ In winter, add an extra $^1/_2$ cup tomatoes and omit the capsicum, as they are then at their most expensive.

Cook's Tips

▶ Putting milk and breadcrumbs into mince mixtures helps keep the mixtures moist. Normally this job is done by the fat but without fat, mince can be dry so use the breadcrumb rule.

▶ Use a heatproof plastic bag like a freezer bag for the grilled capsicum. A standard plastic bag may melt with the intense heat. If you do not have freezer bags, use a plastic container with a lid you do not seal down tightly, so the steam can escape.

Chicken in Thyme Broth

4 teaspoons olive oil

320g boneless chicken pieces, no skin or fat

4 cloves garlic, crushed but not peeled

2 cups sliced spring onions

2 cups thickly sliced or quartered mushrooms

1 cup chopped fresh tomatoes

$\frac{1}{2}$ cup chicken stock, hot

1 sprig fresh thyme

4 cups cooked couscous, hot

Pepper to season

Fresh thyme sprigs to garnish

1. Heat the oil in a frying pan and brown the chicken pieces well. Add the garlic and cook for 1 to 2 minutes.

2. Transfer the chicken to a covered casserole dish and add the spring onions, mushrooms, tomatoes, hot stock and one thyme sprig. Cook at 180°C for 40 to 45 minutes until the chicken is tender.

3. Serve the chicken with its thin juice over hot couscous, seasoned with pepper and garnished with thyme.

Microwave Method

1. Follow recipe step 1.

2. Transfer the chicken and garlic to a microwave-safe dish and add the spring onions, mushrooms, tomatoes, hot stock and thyme.

3. Cover and cook on 70% power for 15 minutes. Leave for 5 minutes. Serve over hot couscous, seasoned with pepper and garnished with thyme.

Cook's Tip

▶ Couscous is now readily available in supermarkets and it makes a refreshing alternative to rice and potatoes. Follow the packet directions for reconstituting but use stock, not just water, to give lots of flavour, otherwise it can be bland. If using stock powder, add 50 Optional Kilojoules for every teaspoon of stock powder or small stock cube used.

SERVES 4

EACH SERVE PROVIDES:
$2\frac{1}{2}$ Vegetable, 1 Fat,
2 Protein, 2 Bread,
5 Optional Kilojoules.
PER SERVE:
8g Fat, 14g Dietary Fibre.

Chicken in Thyme Broth.

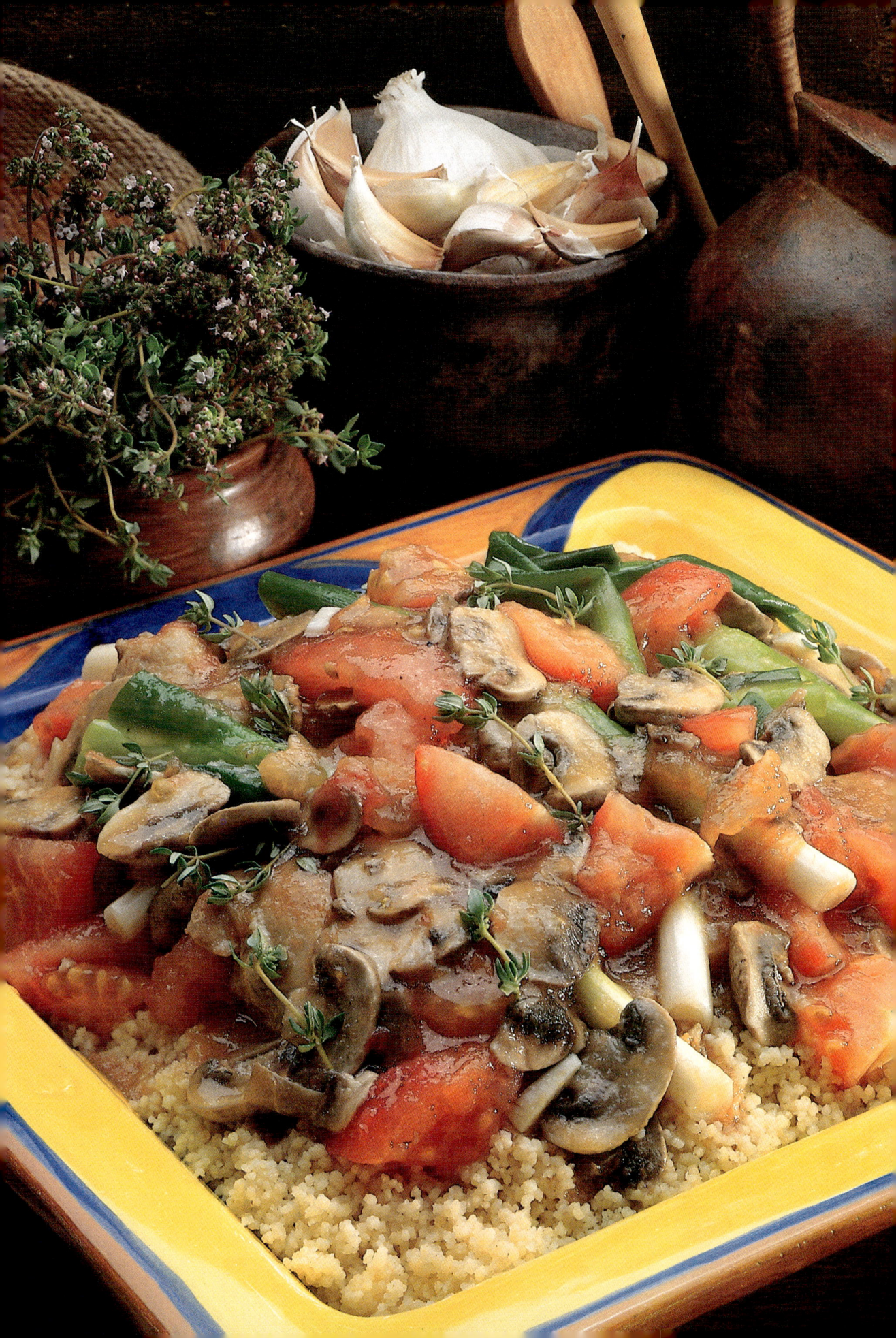

Citrus Chicken

¹/₂ cup
lime or lemon juice

360g chicken breast,
no skin or bone

Grated rind each ¹/₂ lime
or lemon, and ¹/₂ orange

¹/₄ cup orange juice

1¹/₂ tablespoons whole-
grain mustard

1 cup natural low-fat
plain yoghurt

¹/₄ cup water

8 fresh basil leaves,
chopped

Pepper to season

¹/₂ cup chopped
spring onions

1¹/₂ cups diced zucchini

4 cups cooked
jasmine rice, hot

1 orange, segmented
(see Cook's Tip)

1. Sprinkle half the lime juice over the chicken. Grill the chicken under a moderate heat for 12 to 15 minutes until tender, basting regularly with the lime juice. Leave for about 5 minutes before cutting into small pieces.

2. Combine the remaining lime juice, lime rind, orange rind, orange juice, mustard, yoghurt, water and basil. Mix well and season with pepper.

3. Toss the spring onions and zucchini in a frying pan with 2 to 3 tablespoons water until softened and just cooked. Add the chicken and yoghurt mixture, being careful not to let the mixture boil.

4. Serve on four plates over hot jasmine rice and garnished with equal quantities of the orange segments.

Microwave Method

1. Follow the recipe steps 1 and 2.

2. Put the spring onions and zucchini into a microwave-safe bowl. Cover and cook on 100% power for 3 minutes. Add the chicken and yogurt mixture, cover and cook on 70% power for 4 minutes until hot.

3. Serve over hot rice, garnished with orange segments.

Cook's Tip

▶ To segment an orange: cut the peel and pith from the orange. Holding the orange in your hand and using a small paring knife, cut down each side of the membrane on a slight 'V' angle so that each segment will fall out easily. It is a much nicer way to present oranges rather than sliced into rounds or diced.

SERVES 4

EACH SERVE PROVIDES:
¹/₂ Fruit, 1 Vegetable,
2 Protein, 2 Bread, ¹/₂ Milk,
75 Optional Kilojoules.
PER SERVE:
3g Fat, 4¹/₂g Dietary Fibre.

Chicken and Pork Sausages

1 cup finely chopped leeks

200g lean minced pork

200g minced chicken

3 teaspoons wholegrain mustard

1¹/₂ slices wholemeal bread, crumbed

1 teaspoon fresh sage

Pepper to season

SPICY PLUM SAUCE

1 teaspoon chopped fresh ginger

¹/₄ teaspoon chilli powder

¹/₂ teaspoon sesame oil

1 cup cooked plums, chopped and pitted

1 tablespoon chopped fresh coriander

1. Cook the leeks with a splash of water in a covered microwave-safe dish for 4 minutes on 100% power. Leave for 1 minute and drain well. Alternatively heat 3 tablespoons of water in a frying pan and cook the leeks for 3 to 4 minutes.

2. Mix the leeks, minced pork and chicken, mustard, breadcrumbs and sage together. Season with pepper.

3. With wet hands, shape the meat mixture into eight even-sized sausages.

4. Grill the sausages under a high heat for about 8 minutes, turning frequently. They should be golden brown and well cooked.

5. To prepare the sauce, put the ginger, chilli and sesame oil into a small microwave-safe dish, cover and cook on 100% power for about 1¹/₂ minutes. Combine with the chopped plums and coriander. Serve warm or cold over the sausages.

Cook's Tips

▶ If you do not have plums, tamarillos are also delicious with these homemade sausages.

▶ This dish goes well with seasonal vegetables.

SERVES 4

EACH SERVE PROVIDES:
¹/₂ Fruit, ¹/₂ Vegetable,
2¹/₂ Protein, ¹/₄ Bread,
60 Optional Kilojoules.
PER SERVE:
3g Fat, 3¹/₂g Dietary Fibre.

Chicken in Dijon Sauce

4 teaspoons olive oil

360g boneless chicken pieces, no skin or fat

1 cup sliced onion

125 mL white wine

1 tablespoon plain flour

1 tablespoon Dijon mustard

1 cup chicken stock

50g light sour cream

2 tablespoons chopped fresh tarragon or 1 teaspoon dried

Pepper to season

1. Heat the oil in a frying pan and cook the chicken pieces over a moderately high heat until the chicken begins to colour slightly.

2. Add the onion and wine, and reduce the liquid by half.

3. Mix together the flour, mustard, stock and sour cream, and pour over the chicken.

4. Transfer the chicken and sauce to an ovenproof dish and bake at 180°C for 35–40 minutes until tender. Add the tarragon and pepper.

Microwave Method

1. Follow the recipe steps 1, 2 and 3.

2. Transfer the chicken and sauce to a microwave-safe dish.

3. Cook on 70% power for 10 minutes and then stand for 3 minutes. Add the tarragon and season with pepper.

Cook's Tips

▶ Chicken thigh portions have been used for most of the chicken dishes as the meat has more flavour and will stay moist when cooked. They are often cheaper too, making them an excellent choice.

▶ Be sure to use only a mild mustard for this dish.

▶ Serve with rice and green vegetables or salad.

SERVES 4

EACH SERVE PROVIDES:
$^1/_2$ Vegetable, 1 Fat,
2 Protein,
240 Optional Kilojoules.
PER SERVE:
$9^1/_2$g Fat, 1g Dietary Fibre.

*Chicken in Dijon Sauce
served with rice and green vegetables.*

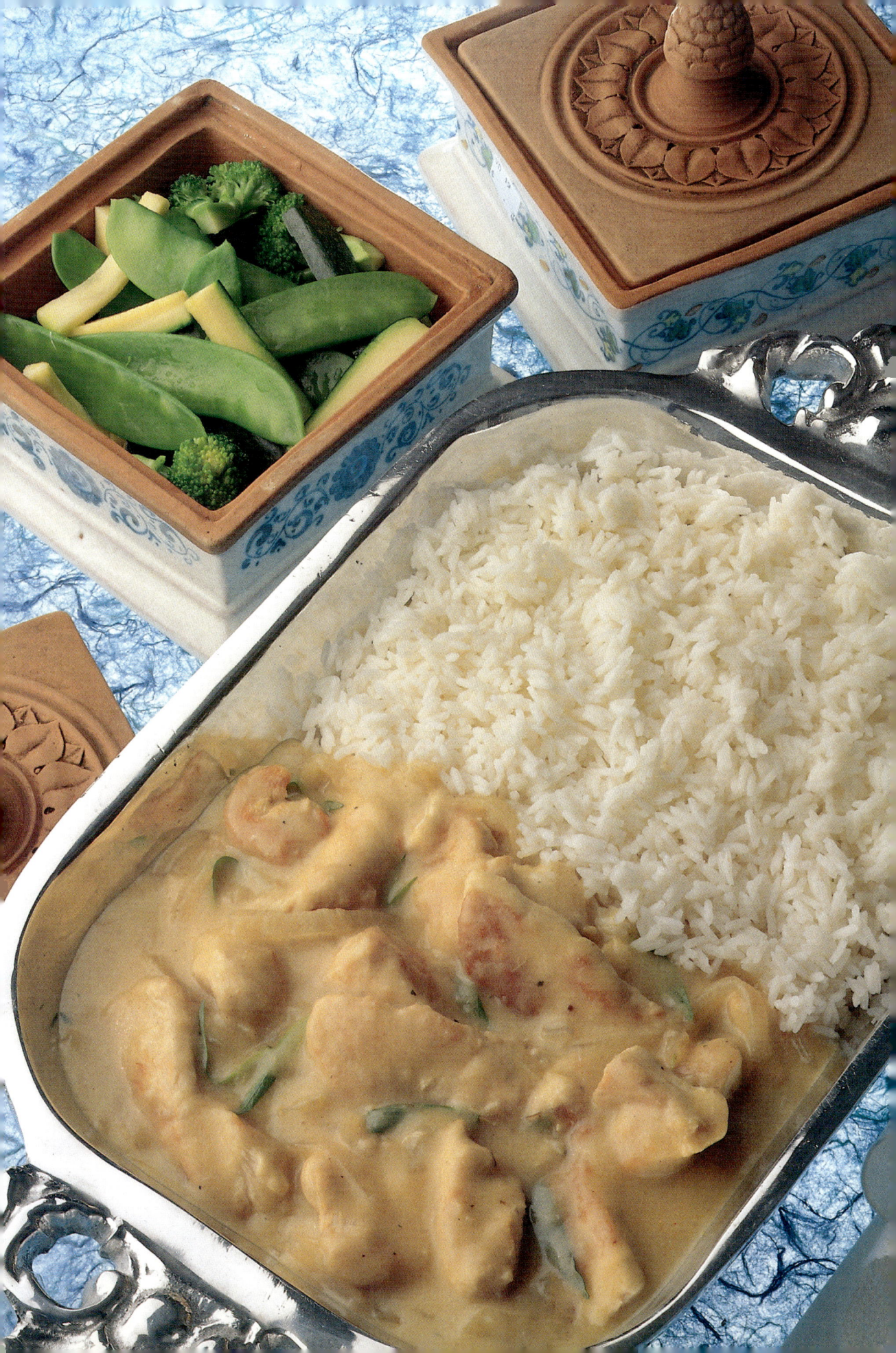

Italian Style Lamb

320g lean lamb steaks

2 teaspoons olive oil

1 clove garlic, crushed

1 cup finely chopped onion

$1/2$ cup tomato paste

$1/2$ cup each diced red and green capsicum

2 cups chopped tomatoes (fresh or canned)

$1^1/2$ cups diced zucchini

20g sliced stuffed olives

2 teaspoons chopped fresh rosemary or $1/2$ teaspoon dried

Pepper to season

4 cups cooked spiral pasta, hot

1. Grill the lamb steaks under a high heat until they brown on both sides. Leave for a few minutes before cutting them into small slices.

2. Heat the oil in a saucepan and cook the garlic and onion for 2 to 3 minutes until just soft. Add the tomato paste and cook for 2 minutes, stirring until the paste darkens a little.

3. Add the capsicum, tomatoes, zucchini, olives, rosemary and lamb. Simmer for 5 to 8 minutes until all the ingredients are just cooked.

4. Season with pepper, toss through hot cooked pasta and serve immediately.

Microwave Method

1. Grill the lamb as above.

2. Put the garlic and onion into a microwave-safe bowl. Cover and cook on 100% power for 3 minutes. Add the tomato paste and capsicum, and microwave for a further 3 minutes on 100% power.

3. Add the chopped tomatoes, cover the dish and return to the microwave for 3 minutes on 100% power.

4. Stir in the zucchini, olives, rosemary and lamb. Cover and cook again for 8 minutes on 70% power. Leave for 2 minutes before seasoning with pepper and tossing though the hot pasta.

NOTE: If using the microwave method, delete $1/2$ Fat Selection per serve.

SERVES 4

EACH SERVE PROVIDES:
3 Vegetable, $1/2$ Fat,
2 Protein, 2 Bread,
10 Optional Kilojoules.
PER SERVE:
$6^1/2$g Fat, $5^1/2$g Dietary Fibre.

Lamb with Black Bean Sauce

450g lean lamb steaks

2 tablespoons
black bean sauce

2 tablespoons Chinese
rice wine vinegar or
cider vinegar

2 teaspoons olive oil

1 chilli,
chopped and seeded

1 clove garlic, crushed

2 teaspoons
chopped fresh ginger

1 1/2 cups finely chopped
leeks

1 cup diced red capsicum

1 1/2 cups broccoli florets

1 cup drained canned
sliced baby corn

3 cups cooked
cellophane noodles

1. Grill the lamb steaks under a hot grill until they are well browned but still pink inside. Leave for 3 to 4 minutes before cutting into thin strips.

2. In a bowl, mix the lamb and any meat juices, black bean sauce and rice wine vinegar. Marinate while preparing the remaining ingredients.

3. In a frying pan, heat the oil and cook the chilli, garlic and ginger over a moderate heat for about 2 minutes.

4. Add the leeks and capsicum and toss for a few more minutes until the vegetables begin to wilt. Add the broccoli and corn with a splash of water, cover and steam for about 2 minutes.

5. Add the lamb and black bean mix, and toss through all the ingredients. Serve over hot noodles.

Microwave Method

1. Follow the recipe steps 1 and 2.

2. Put the chilli, garlic, ginger, chilli, leeks and capsicum in a microwave-safe dish with a good splash of water. Cover and cook on 100% power for 3 minutes. Add the broccoli and baby corn, cover and cook for a further 2 minutes.

3. Toss all ingredients and reheat on 100% power for about 2 minutes before serving over noodles.

NOTE: If using the microwave method, delete 1/2 Fat Selection for each serve and reduce Fat to 5g per serve.

Variation

▶ Use fish, chicken or beef instead of lamb.

SERVES 4

EACH SERVE PROVIDES:
2 Vegetable, 1/2 Fat,
3 Protein, 2 Bread,
55 Optional Kilojoules.
PER SERVE:
7g Fat, 6g Dietary Fibre.

Chicken Hot Pot

4 teaspoons olive oil

1 clove garlic, crushed

1 cup finely chopped onion

1 cup finely chopped celery

1 cup finely chopped carrot

360g boneless chicken thigh pieces, no skin or fat

3 teaspoons cornflour

1 cup chicken stock

50g light sour cream

3 teaspoons chopped fresh tarragon or thyme

Freshly ground black pepper to season

400g peeled, whole cooked potatoes

Fresh tarragon or thyme to garnish

1. Heat the oil in a large, covered frying pan and cook the garlic, onion, celery and carrot for 5 minutes until they are softened but not brown. Add the chicken and brown well.

2. Mix the cornflour, stock and sour cream, and pour over. Season with tarragon and pepper.

3. Simmer covered for 30 minutes until the chicken is tender. Transfer to a serving dish.

4. Slice the potatoes and arrange them on top of the chicken. Brown under the grill until hot and golden. Serve garnished with tarragon.

Microwave Method

1. Put the garlic, onion, celery and carrot into a microwave-safe dish. Cover loosely with plastic wrap and cook on 100% power for 4 minutes. Set aside.

2. Arrange the chicken portions in an even layer in a deep microwave-safe dish that is also grill-proof (glass or crockery). Scatter over the cooked vegetables and tarragon.

3. Mix the cornflour, stock and sour cream and pour over the chicken. Season with pepper.

4. Cover and cook on 70% power for 10 minutes. Slice the potatoes and arrange in a layer on top of the chicken. Cover and cook on 100% power for 2 minutes.

NOTE: If using the microwave method, delete 1 Fat Selection for each serve and reduce Fat to $5\frac{1}{2}$g per serve.

SERVES 4

EACH SERVE PROVIDES:
$1\frac{1}{2}$ Vegetable, 1 Fat,
2 Protein, 1 Bread,
225 Optional Kilojoules.
PER SERVE:
$9\frac{1}{2}$g Fat, 4g Dietary Fibre.

Chicken Hot Pot (top);
Rack of Lamb with Pumpkin Sauce (page 60)
served with vegetables and wholemeal pasta.

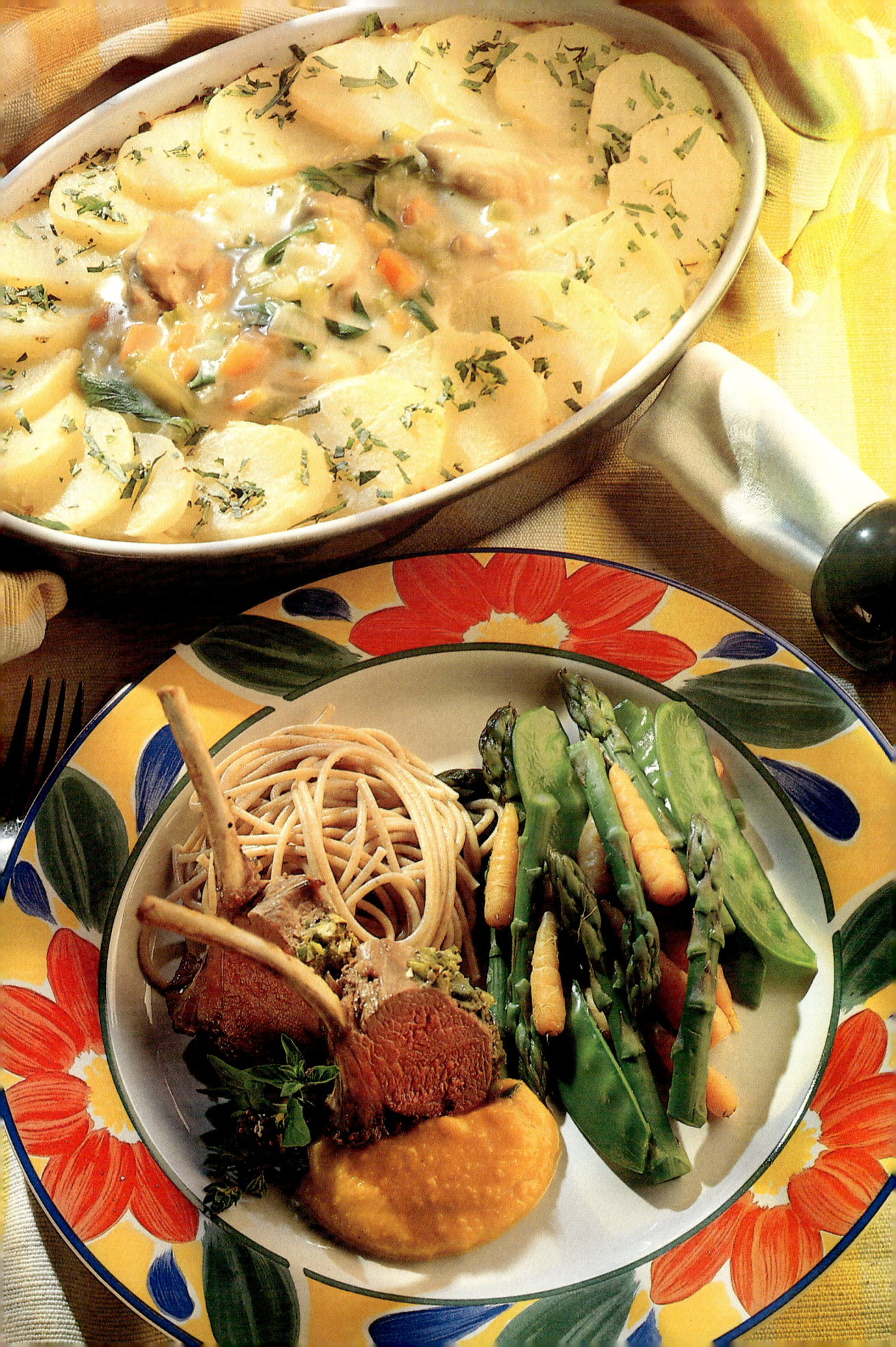

Rack of Lamb with Pumpkin Sauce

LAMB

1 rack lamb with about 8-10 chops

$^1/_2$ cup minced spring onions

2 teaspoons poly-unsaturated margarine

1 teaspoon each ground ginger and black pepper

SAUCE

1 teaspoon vegetable oil

$^1/_2$ cup diced onion

1 teaspoon curry powder

$^1/_2$ cup chicken stock

1 cup soft pumpkin purée

50g light sour cream or cream cheese

1. Trim the lamb of any fat and sinew or silver skin. If this is left on when the lamb cooks, it will tighten and cause the lamb to twist.

2. Mix the spring onions, margarine, ginger and pepper, and spread evenly over the lamb.

3. Bake the lamb on a rack at 190°C for 30 to 35 minutes. Leave for 5 minutes before carving. This will give you medium rare lamb. If you would like it cooked a little more, add an extra 7 to 8 minutes cooking time.

4. To prepare the sauce, heat the oil in a frying pan and cook the onion and curry powder over a moderate heat until the onion softens. Add the stock, pumpkin purée and light sour cream.

5. Blend or process the mixture until smooth. Serve hot with 60g sliced lamb.

Cook's Tips

▶ The pumpkin purée needs to be soft, otherwise add more chicken stock and remember to count the extra Optional Kilojoules.

▶ Serve this dish with steamed green vegetables and wholemeal pasta.

SERVES 4

EACH SERVE PROVIDES:
1 Vegetable, $^1/_2$ Fat,
2 Protein,
150 Optional Kilojoules.
PER SERVE:
12g Fat, 1g Dietary Fibre.

Pictured page 59.

Minted Orange Lamb

4x100g lean
lamb loin chops

1 orange, peeled
and segmented

MARINADE

1 tablespoon Weight
Watchers marmalade
(preferably orange)

2 tablespoons
orange juice

$1/2$ teaspoon
cracked pepper

1 tablespoon
chopped fresh mint

1. Use a sharp knife to cut the meat from the bone, taking care to remove the meat from both sides. Roll up the chops into a circle and secure with string. Put in an oven-proof casserole dish with a lid.

2. To prepare the marinade, mix the marmalade, orange juice, pepper and mint. Pour over the chops and chill in the refrigerator for 1 hour.

3. Cook the chops under a hot grill for about 5 minutes on each side. Baste with any remaining marinade.

4. Remove string from the lamb. Arrange the orange segments over the lamb.

Cook's Tip

▶ Serve with vegetables or salad.

SERVES 4

EACH SERVE PROVIDES:
$1/4$ Fruit, 2 Protein,
25 Optional Kilojoules
(if ordinary marmalade is
used, then count 70 kJ).
PER SERVE:
4g Fat, 1g Dietary Fibre.

Chilli Lamb and Noodles

320g lamb steaks

6 sun-dried tomatoes
(not packed in oil)

1 cup snow peas

1 teaspoon olive oil

2 red chillies

1 cup finely chopped
onion

1½ cups finely
sliced celery

1½ cups diced
red capsicum

60 mL white wine

¼ cup vegetable stock

2 teaspoons cornflour

2 tablespoons
chopped fresh basil

4 cups cooked pasta
of your choice, hot

1. Grill the lamb steaks on both sides until they are well browned, but still pink in the middle. Leave for 3 to 4 minutes before slicing into very thin strips.

2. Pour ¼ cup boiling water over the sun-dried tomatoes and leave for 5 minutes to swell. Drain, reserving the water and slice the tomatoes into thin strips.

3. Trim and blanch the snow peas in boiling water or in the microwave.

4. Heat the oil in a large frying pan and cook the chillies, onion and celery for about 5 minutes over a moderate heat. Add the capsicum and cook for 2 to 3 minutes.

5. Blend the wine, stock, cornflour, reserved tomato liquid and basil. Pour into the pan with the lamb and all the vegetables. Simmer only until the sauce thickens and warms through. Toss through hot pasta and serve.

Microwave Method

1. Follow the recipe steps 1, 2 and 3.

2. Put the chillies, onion, and celery in a large microwave-safe dish with a splash of water and cover. Cook on 100% power for 4 minutes.

3. Add the capsicum, cover and cook for a further 2 minutes on 100% power.

4. Combine the reserved tomato liquid with the white wine, stock and cornflour, and stir into the cooked vegetables. Add the lamb, basil and tomato slices.

5. Cover and cook on 100% power for 3 minutes. Add the snow peas and cover. Leave for 2 to 3 minutes before tossing through the hot pasta and serving.

NOTE: If using the microwave method, delete 43 Optional Kilojoules for each serve and reduce Fat to 4g per serve.

SERVES 4

EACH SERVE PROVIDES:
3½ Vegetable, 2 Protein,
2 Bread,
70 Optional Kilojoules.
PER SERVE:
5g Fat, 7½g Dietary Fibre.

Chilli Lamb and Noodles (rear);
Steak and Crispy Potato Cakes (page 64)
served with broccoli.

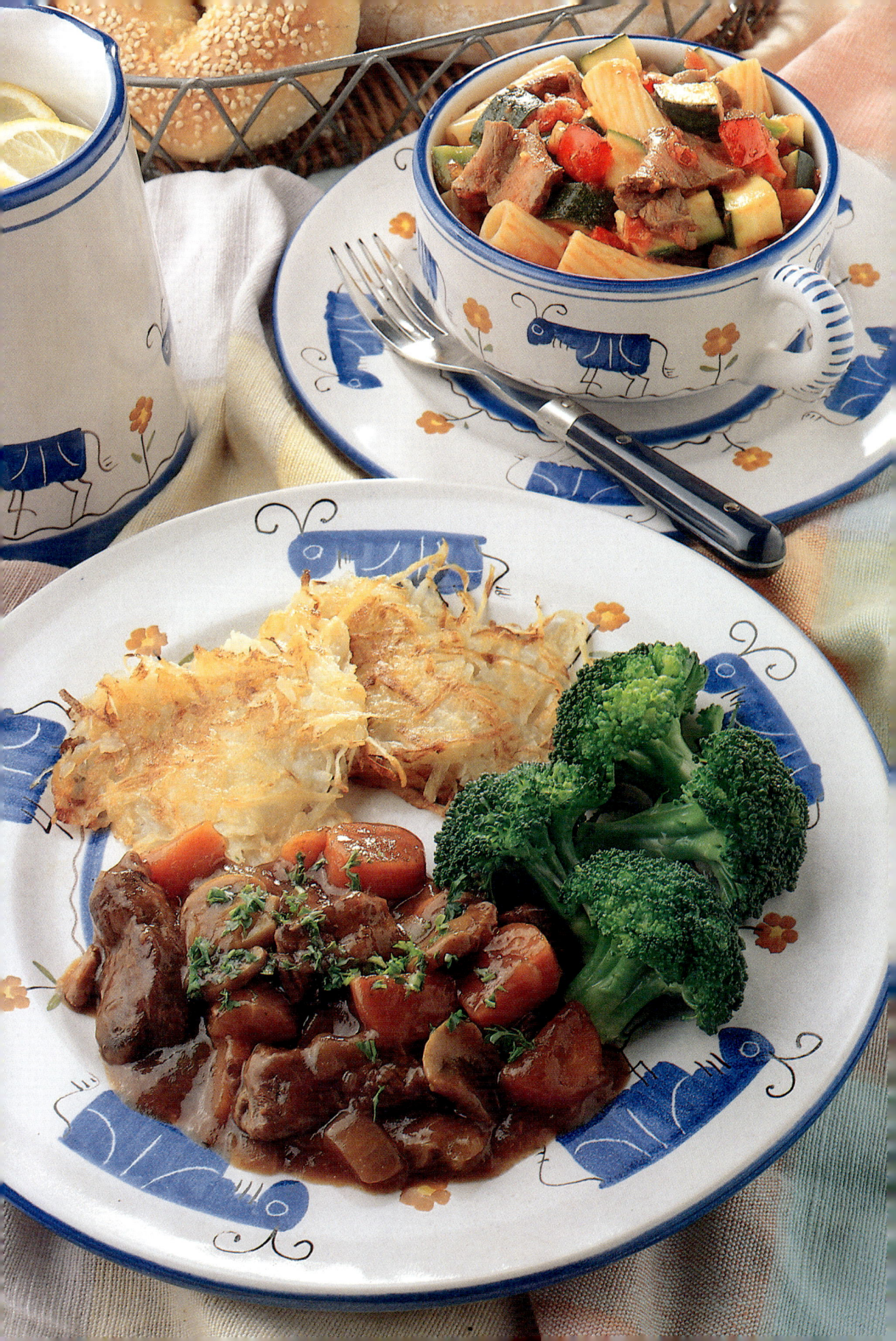

Steak and Crispy Potato Cakes

320g lean blade steak

4 teaspoons vegetable oil

1 clove garlic, crushed

1 cup chopped onion

1 cup chopped carrot

$^1/_2$ cup tomato paste

125 mL red wine

$1^1/_4$ cups beef stock

1 bouquet garni

2 cups finely sliced mushrooms

1 tablespoon cornflour

Ground black pepper to season

1–2 tablespoons chopped fresh parsley to garnish

CRISPY POTATO CAKES

700g grated raw potato

1 cup grated raw parsnips

Pepper to season

1. Grill the meat under a high heat until it browns well on both sides. Leave to stand for 10 minutes before cutting into 2cm pieces.

2. In a frying pan, heat the oil and cook the garlic, onion and carrot for about 5 minutes until they are soft but not brown. Add the tomato paste and cook, stirring until the paste darkens a little. Stir in the red wine, beef stock, bouquet garni and beef.

3. Transfer to a casserole dish and bake at 180°C for about 1 hour until the meat is tender. Add the mushrooms and cornflour mixed with a little water. Cook for a further 10 minutes. Season with pepper, and garnish with the parsley before serving.

4. To prepare the potato cakes, squeeze out any excess moisture from the potatoes. Mix the potatoes and parsnips with pepper to season.

5. Divide into eight equal portions and mould each one into a 10cm diameter cake. Place on a foil-lined baking tray. Bake at 220°C for 15 minutes. Turn and cook for a further 5 minutes. Serves two cakes per person.

Microwave Method

1. Prepare the meat as above.

2. Put the garlic, onion and carrot into a microwave-safe dish with a splash of water. Cover and cook on 100% power for 4 minutes.

3. Stir in the tomato paste, wine, stock, bouquet garni and meat. Cover and cook on 100% power for 3 minutes. Lower the power to 70% and cook for 15 minutes.

4. Add the mushrooms and pepper. Cover and cook on 50% power for 10 minutes until the meat is tender. Prepare potato cakes, follow the recipe steps 4 and 5.

5. Blend the cornflour with a little extra water and stir into the casserole. Leave for 10 minutes to thicken.

6. Garnish with parsley and serve two potato cakes per person.

NOTE: If using the microwave method, delete 1 Fat Selection for each serve and reduce Fat to $4^1/_2$g per serve.

SERVES 4

EACH SERVE PROVIDES:
$2^1/_2$ Vegetable, 1 Fat,
2 Protein, 2 Bread,
65 Optional Kilojoules.
PER SERVE:
$9^1/_2$g Fat, $6^1/_2$g Dietary Fibre.

Pictured page 63.

Spicy Hamburgers

1 slice wholemeal bread, crumbed

¹/₄ cup skim milk

320g minced pork

1 tablespoon dark low-salt soy sauce

3 cloves garlic, crushed

1 teaspoon minced fresh ginger

¹/₂ cup grated carrot

¹/₂ cup minced spring onions

Pepper to season

4x60g hamburger rolls

1. In a bowl, mix the breadcrumbs with the milk. Leave for about 5 minutes.

2. Mix in the pork, soy sauce, garlic, ginger, carrot, spring onions and pepper.

3. Mould into four even-sized patties and cook under a hot grill for 5 minutes on each side.

4. Serve each meat patty on a hamburger bun.

Cook's Tips

▶ The grated carrot in this mixture adds some colour to the finished hamburger.

▶ Serve with salad ingredients of your choice.

SERVES 4

EACH SERVE PROVIDES:
¹/₂ Vegetable, 2 Protein,
2¹/₄ Bread,
25 Optional Kilojoules.
PER SERVE:
3g Fat, 3¹/₂g Dietary Fibre.

Ham Jambalaya

¹/₂ teaspoon each cayenne pepper, white pepper, mustard powder and garlic powder

¹/₄ teaspoon each black pepper, dried thyme and cumin

2 bay leaves

4 teaspoons vegetable oil

1 cup each chopped onion, celery and green capsicum

360g diced lean ham

160g long-grain rice

1¹/₂ cups chicken stock

2¹/₂ cups chopped fresh tomatoes

¹/₂ cup tomato paste

Fresh oregano sprigs to garnish

1 In a bowl, mix together the cayenne, white pepper, mustard powder, garlic powder, black pepper, thyme and cumin. Crunch the bay leaves finely and add. Set aside.

2 Heat the oil in a heavy based pan and cook the chopped onion, celery, capsicum and diced ham over a moderate heat for about 5 minutes.

3 Add the spice mixture and cook for 1 minute.

4 Stir in the rice, stock, tomatoes and tomato paste, and bring to the boil. Lower the heat and simmer gently for about 20 minutes until the rice is well cooked. Serve in large bowls, garnished with oregano.

Variation

▶ Use chicken, pork or seafood instead of the ham if desired. You will need to alter the Selections per serve accordingly.

Cook's Tip

▶ Serve with bowls of green vegetables or a crisp salad.

SERVES 4

EACH SERVE PROVIDES:
3 Vegetable, 1 Fat,
3 Protein, 2 Bread,
25 Optional Kilojoules.
PER SERVE:
8¹/₂g Fat, 3¹/₂g Dietary Fibre.

Ham Jambalaya.

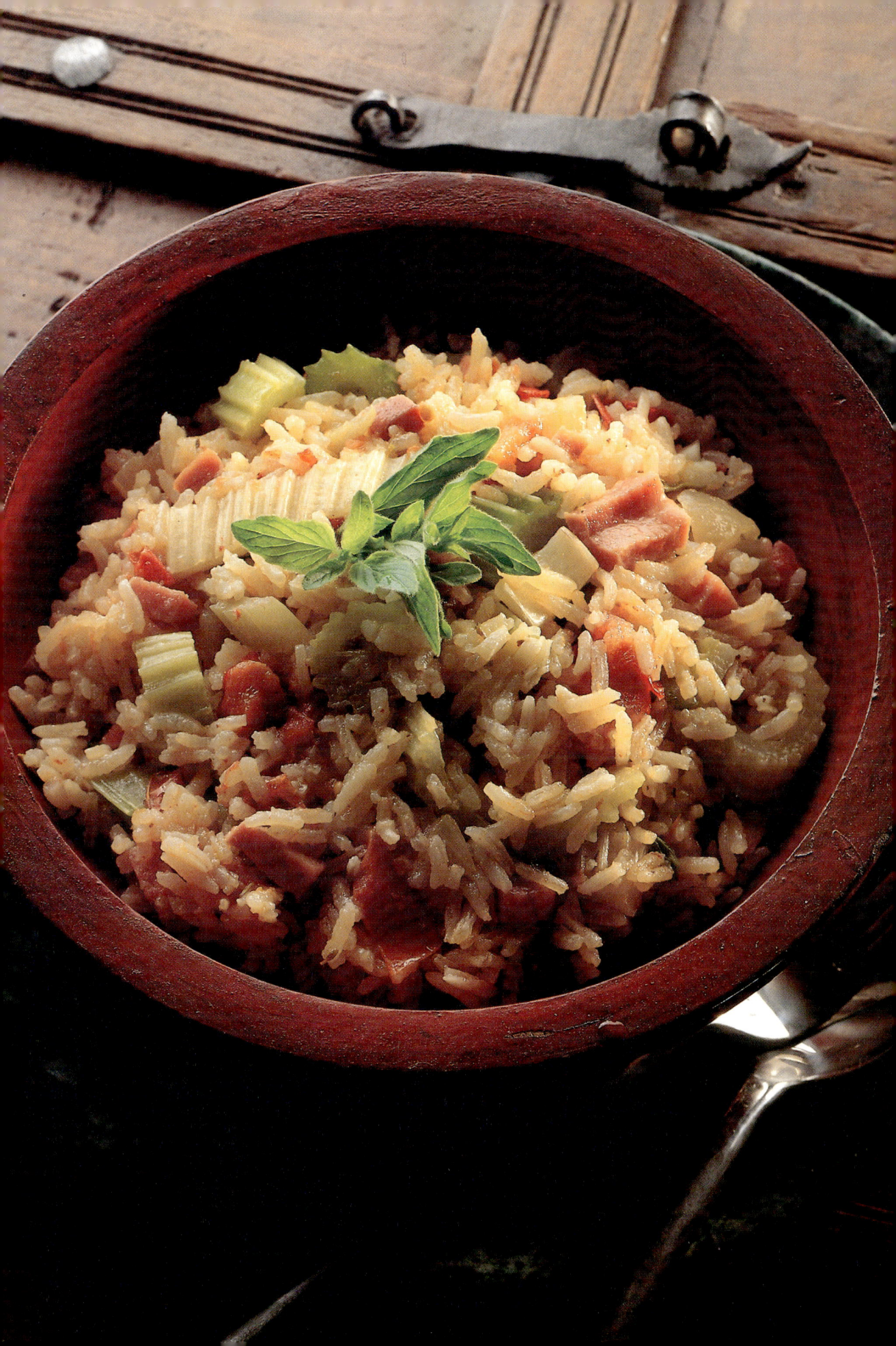

Ham and Asparagus Pasta

2 cups diced
fresh asparagus

2 cups chicken stock

1 cup thinly sliced leeks

1 cup sliced celery

120g shredded ham

80g Brie cheese, sliced

25g light cream cheese

2 teaspoons cornflour

4 cups cooked
spaghetti, hot

Chopped fresh parsley or
tarragon to garnish

1. Blanch the asparagus and drain well.

2. Simmer the asparagus, stock, leeks, celery and ham in a large saucepan for about 3 minutes.

3. Add the Brie and cream cheese, and stir as they melt.

4. Mix the cornflour with a little water and stir in. Cook until the sauce thickens.

5. Toss the sauce over cooked pasta and serve garnished with fresh parsley.

Cook's Tip

▶ This dish tastes good served with spinach or tomato pasta, so do try them.

SERVES 4

EACH SERVE PROVIDES:
2 Vegetable, 2 Protein,
2 Bread,
100 Optional Kilojoules.
PER SERVE:
9g Fat, 5g Dietary Fibre.

Pork Meatballs in Mushroom Sauce

1 slice wholemeal bread, crumbed

$^1/_2$ cup skim milk

320g minced pork

2 hard-cooked eggs, sieved or finely chopped

1 tablespoon chopped capers

1 tablespoon chopped fresh dill or 1 teaspoon dried

SAUCE

4 teaspoons vegetable oil

1 cup sliced onion

2 cups sliced mushrooms

1 cup skim milk

$1^1/_2$ tablespoons cornflour

$^1/_2$ cup chicken stock

1 tablespoon chopped fresh dill or 2 teaspoons dried

1. In a bowl, mix the breadcrumbs with the milk. Leave for 10 minutes.
2. Add the pork, eggs, capers and dill, and mix well.
3. Roll tablespoonfuls into balls and cook under a hot grill, turning to brown all sides evenly.
4. To prepare the sauce, heat the oil in a frying pan and cook the onion and mushrooms until soft but not brown.
5. Mix the skim milk, cornflour and stock, and stir into the pan. Simmer for 3 to 5 minutes until the sauce thickens. Stir through the dill.
6. Toss the meatballs in the sauce and serve.

Variation

▶ If you do not have capers, substitute gherkins or pickled asparagus.

Cook's Tips

▶ Serve these meatballs and sauce over rice.

▶ If you have trouble moulding the mince into balls, try wetting your hands first.

SERVES 4

EACH SERVE PROVIDES:
$1^1/_2$ Vegetable, 1 Fat,
$2^1/_2$ Protein, $^1/_4$ Bread, $^1/_4$ Milk,
130 Optional Kilojoules.
PER SERVE:
10g Fat, 2g Dietary Fibre.

Pork in Cider

80g green or brown lentils
320g lean pork shoulder
2 teaspoons olive oil
1 cup finely chopped onion
1 cup finely chopped celery
1 clove garlic, crushed
2 small apples, sliced
$\frac{1}{2}$ cup cider
$1\frac{1}{2}$ cups chicken stock
2 sprigs fresh thyme
$1\frac{1}{2}$ tablespoons cornflour
1 tablespoon chopped fresh parsley
1 teaspoon chopped fresh thyme or pinch dried to garnish

1. Cook the lentils in boiling water for 30 minutes until tender. Drain well.

2. Dice the pork into 2cm small pieces. Heat the oil in a frying pan and cook the pork over a moderate heat until well browned.

3. Transfer the meat and lentils to a casserole dish. Add the onion, celery, garlic, apples, cider, $1\frac{1}{4}$ cups chicken stock and thyme.

4. Bake at 180°C for 1 hour. Blend the cornflour with the remaining stock and stir in. Cook for a further 5 minutes until thickened. Garnish with parsley and thyme and serve.

Microwave Method

1. Follow the recipe steps 1 and 2.

2. Put the onion, celery and garlic into a microwave-safe container with a splash of water. Cover and cook on 100% power for 4 minutes.

3. Add the apples, cider, $1\frac{1}{4}$ cups stock and thyme. Cover and cook on 100% power for a further 2 to 3 minutes until very hot.

4. Add the pork and lentils. Cover and cook on 70% power for 20–25 minutes until tender. Blend the cornflour with the remaining stock and stir into the meat. Cover and leave for 5 minutes to let the sauce thicken. Garnish with parsley and thyme before serving.

Cook's Tip

▶ Cooked sweet potatoes go really well with this dish. They can be boiled, baked or microwaved until tender.

SERVES 4

EACH SERVE PROVIDES:
$\frac{1}{2}$ Fruit, 1 Vegetable,
$\frac{1}{2}$ Fat, 2 Protein, 1 Bread
(lentils could also be extra Protein)
155 Optional Kilojoules.
PER SERVE:
$4\frac{1}{2}$g Fat, 5g Dietary Fibre.

Pork in Cider (bottom) served with vegetables;
Mexican Beef with Cornmeal (page 72).

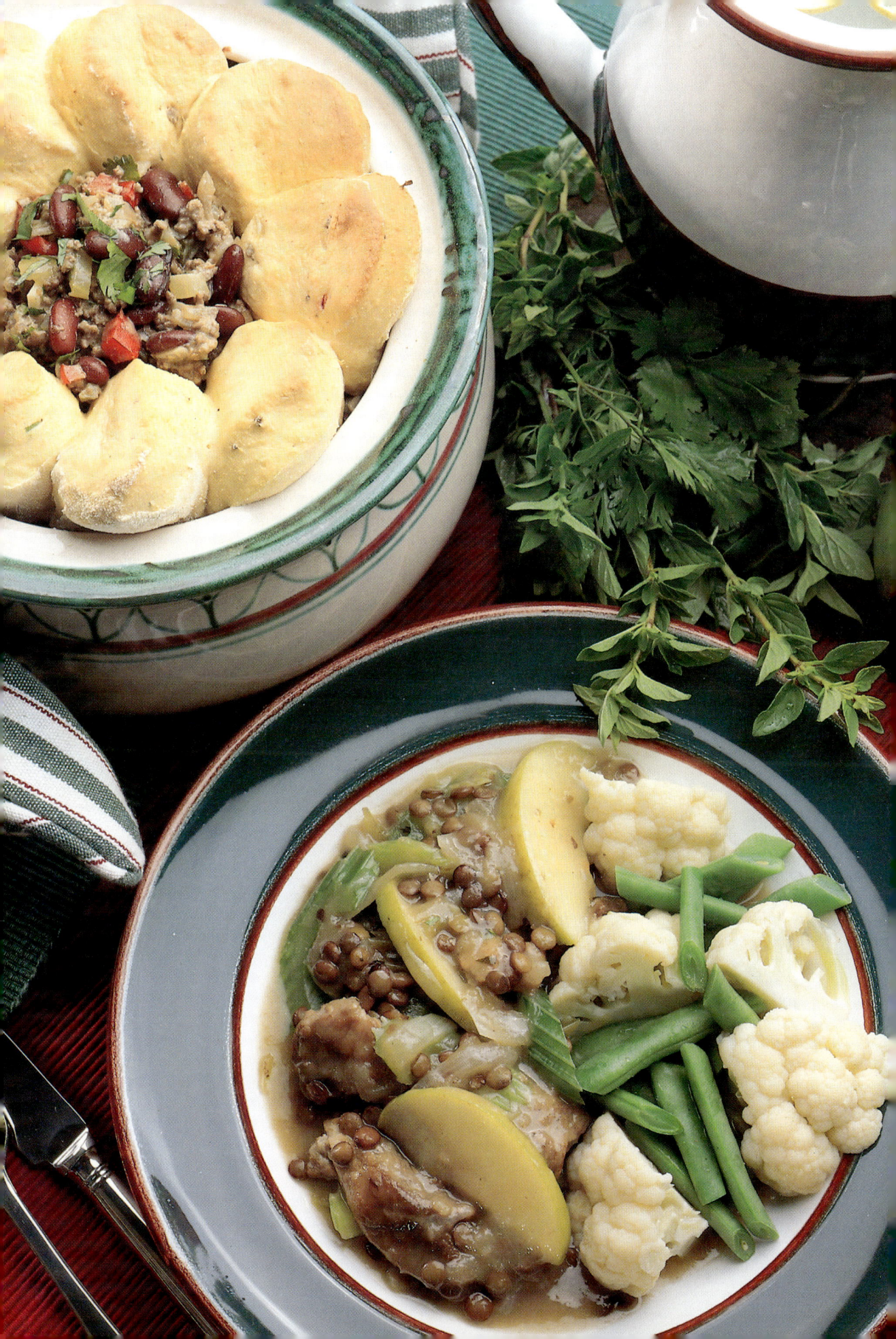

Mexican Beef with Cornmeal

2 teaspoons vegetable oil

1 cup finely chopped onion

1 cup finely chopped celery

1 clove garlic, crushed

1 teaspoon chopped fresh red chilli

240g premium lean minced beef

1 cup diced red capsicum

$^1/_2$ teaspoon cumin

120g cooked red kidney beans

$^1/_2$ cup natural low-fat yoghurt

$^1/_2$ cup beef stock

1 tablespoon chopped fresh coriander

CORNMEAL TOPPING

120g plain flour

40g fine cornmeal

2$^1/_4$ teaspoons baking powder

$^1/_4$ teaspoon each cumin, chilli powder and dried thyme

$^1/_2$ cup skim milk

SERVES 4

EACH SERVE PROVIDES:
$^1/_2$ Fruit, 1$^1/_2$ Vegetable,
$^1/_2$ Fat, 2 Protein,
2 Bread, $^1/_4$ Milk,
50 Optional Kilojoules.
PER SERVE:
6g Fat, 5g Dietary Fibre.

1. Heat the oil in a frying pan and cook the onion, celery, garlic and chilli over a moderate heat for 5 minutes until the onion is soft but not brown.

2. Add the beef and brown well. Add the capsicum, cumin, beans, yoghurt, stock and coriander. Turn into a shallow ovenproof dish and set aside.

3. To prepare the topping, sift the flour, cornmeal, baking powder, cumin, chilli powder and thyme into a bowl. Stir in the milk to form a soft dough.

4. Turn out and knead on a lightly floured board until smooth. Roll out to 1cm thickness and cut into triangles. Arrange around the edge of the beef dish. Brush the dough with milk.

5. Bake at 190°C for 20 minutes until the cornmeal topping is well risen and golden. Serve hot.

Cook's Tips

▶ Accompany with a crisp green salad. A spinach and sprout salad would be great. Add a few pieces of fruit.

▶ Keep a jar of chilli paste in the refrigerator. A touch of chilli will add a lot of flavour to many dishes, without being overpowering or too hot! It also makes for easy use.

Pictured page 71.

Pork Schnitzels with Fennel Sauce

SCHNITZELS

4x80g pork schnitzels

2 teaspoons olive oil

2 cups sliced eggplant

8 fresh basil leaves

Pinch dried oregano or
marjoram

Cracked pepper to season

2 teaspoons olive oil

120g diced potatoes

SAUCE

1½ cups diced
fennel bulb

1 clove garlic, crushed

½ cup diced onion

1 tablespoon plain flour

1½ cups chicken stock

2 tablespoons chopped
fennel fronds

1 teaspoon
wholegrain mustard

Pepper to season

① Place the schnitzels between two dampened sheets of plastic and flatten them with a mallet until they are quite thin. Set aside.

② Heat 2 teaspoons oil in a frying pan and cook the eggplant slices until brown and soft. Leave to cool.

③ Place the four schnitzels on a board and top each with eggplant and basil leaves. Sprinkle with oregano and pepper.

④ Roll up the schnitzels and secure with a toothpick.

⑤ In a pan, heat 2 teaspoons oil and brown the schnitzels. Transfer to a casserole dish.

⑥ To prepare the sauce, add the diced fennel, garlic and onion to the pan and toss until brown. Stir in the flour and toss to coat the vegetables. Pour in the stock and stir until a smooth sauce forms. Pour the sauce over the pork and scatter the potatoes over.

⑦ Cook at 180°C for 45 to 50 minutes until the pork is tender. Stir in the fennel fronds and mustard, and season with pepper before serving.

Microwave Method

① Follow the recipe steps 1 to 6.

② Transfer schnitzels, sauce and potatoes to a microwave-safe dish and cook on 70% power for 5 minutes. Lower the power level to 30% and cook for 20 to 25 minutes.

③ Leave for 5 minutes before stirring in the fennel fronds and mustard. Season with pepper and serve.

Cook's Tip

▶ Fennel bulbs have a mild, sweet, aniseed flavour which is stronger when raw. It adds variety to salads, rice dishes and pasta meals. Use the fronds, the top leafy parts, for final flavouring and garnishing.

SERVES 4

EACH SERVE PROVIDES:
2 Vegetable, 1 Fat,
2 Protein, ½ Bread,
35 Optional Kilojoules.
PER SERVE:
7g Fat, 4g Dietary Fibre.

Steak and Kidney Casserole

320g lean beef

80g kidneys

1 teaspoon vegetable oil

1 cup diced onion

3 cups sliced mushrooms

¼ cup tomato paste

1½ tablespoons
plain flour

2 tablespoons
Worcestershire sauce

1½ cups beef stock

1 teaspoon
cracked pepper

Chopped fresh parsley
to garnish

PASTRY

140g plain flour

20g wheatgerm

30g polyunsaturated
margarine

Cold water

1. Cut the beef into large pieces and grill under a high heat until it browns well.

2. Cut the kidneys in half and trim away the core. Slice the kidneys into thirds.

3. Heat the oil in a frying pan and cook the onion, mushrooms and kidneys over a moderately high heat until the onion softens and the kidneys brown.

4. Stir in the tomato paste and flour, and cook for about 3 minutes. Add the Worcesterhire sauce, stock and pepper. Mix to a smooth sauce.

5. Transfer to a casserole dish with the beef. Cover and bake at 180°C for 1 to 1¼ hours. Leave for 10 minutes before garnishing with parsley. Serve with a pastry wedge.

6. To prepare the pastry, blend or process the flour, wheatgerm and margarine until the mixture resembles fine crumbs. With the motor running, pour sufficient cold water down the feedtube until the mixture forms small beads of dough.

7. Roll out the dough to make a long strip. Fold into thirds and give a quarter turn. Roll and fold once more. Leave the dough to stand for 10 minutes then roll out to a 23cm circle. Mark into eight equal wedges. Transfer to a baking tray lightly coated with non-stick cooking spray.

8. Bake at 220°C for 12 to 15 minutes until well risen and golden in colour.

Microwave Method

1. Follow the recipe steps 1 to 4.

2. Transfer to a microwave-safe dish. Add the meat and cover. Cook on 70% power for 5 minutes, then lower to 30% power for 45 minutes until the meat is tender.

3. Follow steps 6 to 8 to make the pastry.

SERVES 4

EACH SERVE PROVIDES:
2¼ Vegetable, 1½ Fat,
2½ Protein, 2 Bread,
135 Optional Kilojoules.
PER SERVE:
12g Fat, 4g Dietary Fibre.

Steak and Kidney Casserole.

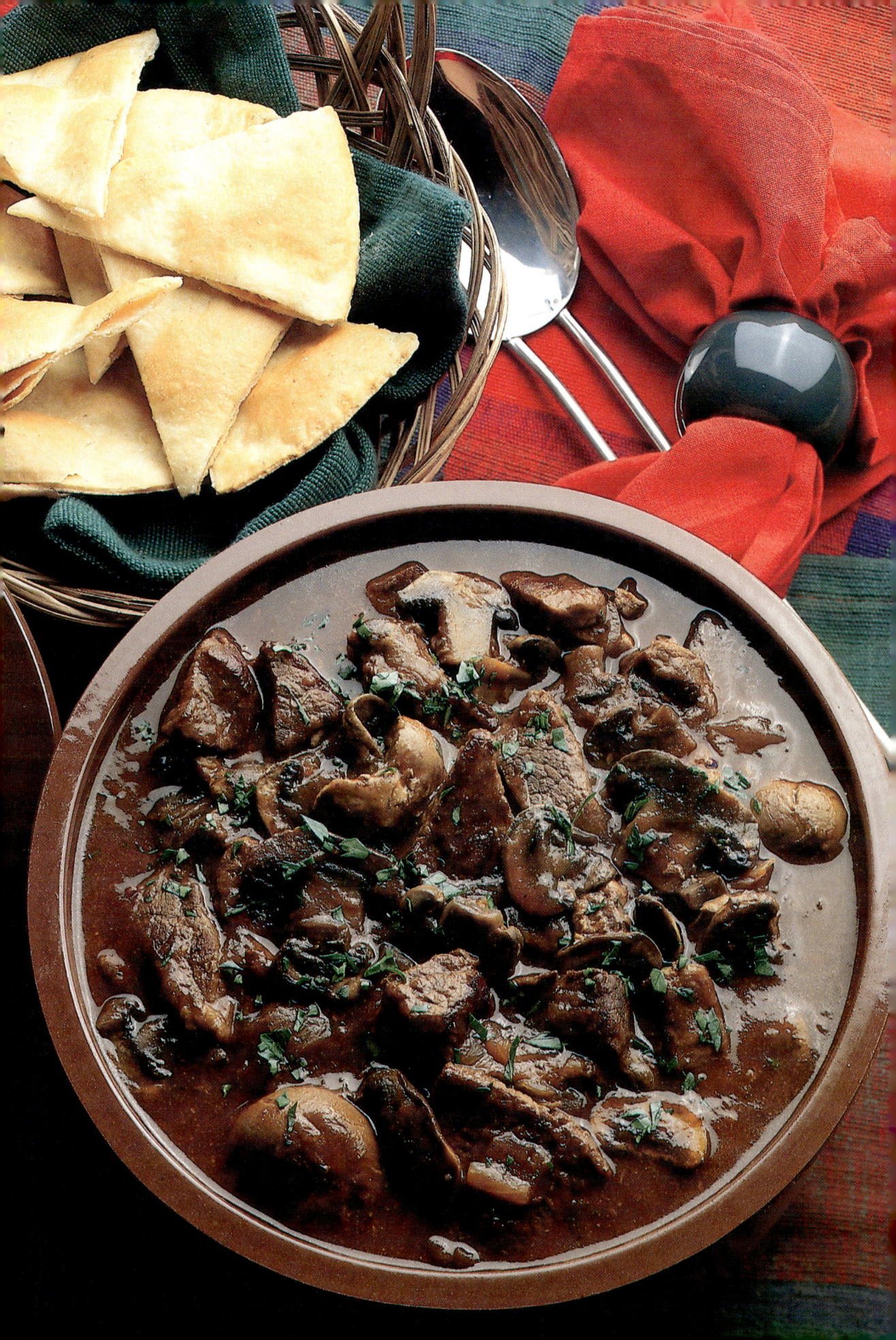

Beef and Pesto Tart

2 slices wholemeal bread, crumbed

$^1/_2$ cup skim milk

320g premium minced beef

1 cup minced spring onions

3 cloves garlic, crushed

$^1/_2$ cup fresh basil, finely chopped

40g grated Parmesan cheese

$^1/_2$ cup cooked barley

Pepper to season

1. In a bowl, mix the breadcrumbs with the milk. Leave for about 5 minutes.

2. Mix in the beef, spring onions, garlic, basil, Parmesan and barley. Season well with pepper.

3. Spread the mixture to a depth of about 1.5cm in a Swiss roll pan. Smooth the top and mark lines with the back of a knife.

4. Bake at 180°C for 30 minutes. Brown under a hot grill for 4 to 5 minutes until the slice is golden and crispy.

Cook's Tips

▶ Serve warm with slices of fresh tomato.

▶ This dish is ideal for a picnic when cut into squares for hamburgers.

SERVES 4

EACH SERVE PROVIDES:
$^1/_2$ Vegetable, $2^1/_2$ Protein,
$^3/_4$ Bread.
45 Optional Kilojoules.
PER SERVE:
7g Fat, $2^1/_2$g Dietary Fibre.

Sesame Beef Salad

450g lean rump steak

1 tablespoon oyster sauce

1 tablespoon
white wine vinegar

1 teaspoon toasted
sesame seeds

1 teaspoon sesame oil

1 clove garlic, crushed

2 teaspoons finely
chopped fresh ginger

2¹/₂ cups broccoli florets

2 cups sliced zucchini

2 cups sliced celery

¹/₂ cup spring onions,
sliced diagonally

4x60g Naan bread

1. Grill the beef on both sides under a hot grill until well browned but still pink inside. Leave for 3 to 4 minutes before slicing the beef into very thin strips.

2. Combine the beef strips, oyster sauce, wine vinegar and sesame seeds, and marinate for 5 to 10 minutes.

3. In a frying pan, heat the sesame oil and cook the garlic and ginger over a moderate heat for about 2 minutes.

4. Add the broccoli, zucchini and a splash of water. Toss until slightly cooked. The water will help steam the vegetables and avoid burning.

5. In a large bowl, combine the beef mixture with the broccoli and zucchini. Mix in the raw celery and spring onions. Serve with Naan bread.

Cook's Tips

▶ The celery and zucchini can be cut into long batons to look more interesting.

▶ Naan bread is an Indian leavened bread which is traditionally baked in a Tandoor or clay oven.

SERVES 4

EACH SERVE PROVIDES:
3¹/₂ Vegetable, ¹/₄ Fat,
3 Protein, 2 Bread,
75 Optional Kilojoules.
PER SERVE:
6¹/₂g Fat, 8g Dietary Fibre.

VEGETARIAN

More and more people today are including vegetarian meals as part of a regular eating plan. With all the different kinds of grains, pulses and legumes available, the options are endless. Look for the newer style grains such as couscous and burghul wheat which have always been available but are now more popular. They go well with all vegetables and many herbs, making for fabulous meatless meals which are tasty, filling and full of vitamins, minerals and fibre.

Mexican Hot Pot

2 teaspoons olive oil
1 cup diced onion
3 cloves garlic, crushed
3 teaspoons chopped mild jalapeño peppers
$\frac{1}{2}$ teaspoon each cumin and ground coriander
1 teaspoon each paprika and pepper
3 cups chopped tomatoes
2 cups corn kernels
200g diced potatoes
1 cup vegetable stock
1 cup sliced green beans
240g cooked kidney beans

1. In a frying pan, heat the oil and cook the onion, garlic, jalapeño peppers, cumin, coriander, paprika and pepper over a moderate heat for about 5 minutes until the onion is soft.

2. Add the tomatoes, corn, potatoes and stock, and simmer for 15 minutes.

3. Add both types of beans and simmer for a further 5 minutes. Serve in large bowls.

Microwave Method

1. In a frying pan, heat the oil and cook the onion to bring out the natural sugars and add flavour.

2. Put in a covered microwave-safe dish and combine the rest of the ingredients, apart from both types of beans. Cook on 100% power for 8 minutes.

3. Add the beans and cook for a further 3 to 4 minutes on 100% power. Leave for 2 minutes before serving.

Cook's Tip

▶ If you do not have any jalapeño peppers, use $\frac{1}{2}$ teaspoon chilli powder or to taste. Jalapeño peppers are available fresh or canned. Be careful if choosing the canned variety, as they are available mild, medium or hot! You will find them in the Mexican section of your supermarket.

SERVES 4

EACH SERVE PROVIDES:
$2\frac{1}{2}$ Vegetable, $\frac{1}{2}$ Fat,
1 Protein, $1\frac{1}{2}$ Bread,
15 Optional Kilojoules.
PER SERVE:
4g Fat, 10g Dietary Fibre.

Mexican Hot Pot.

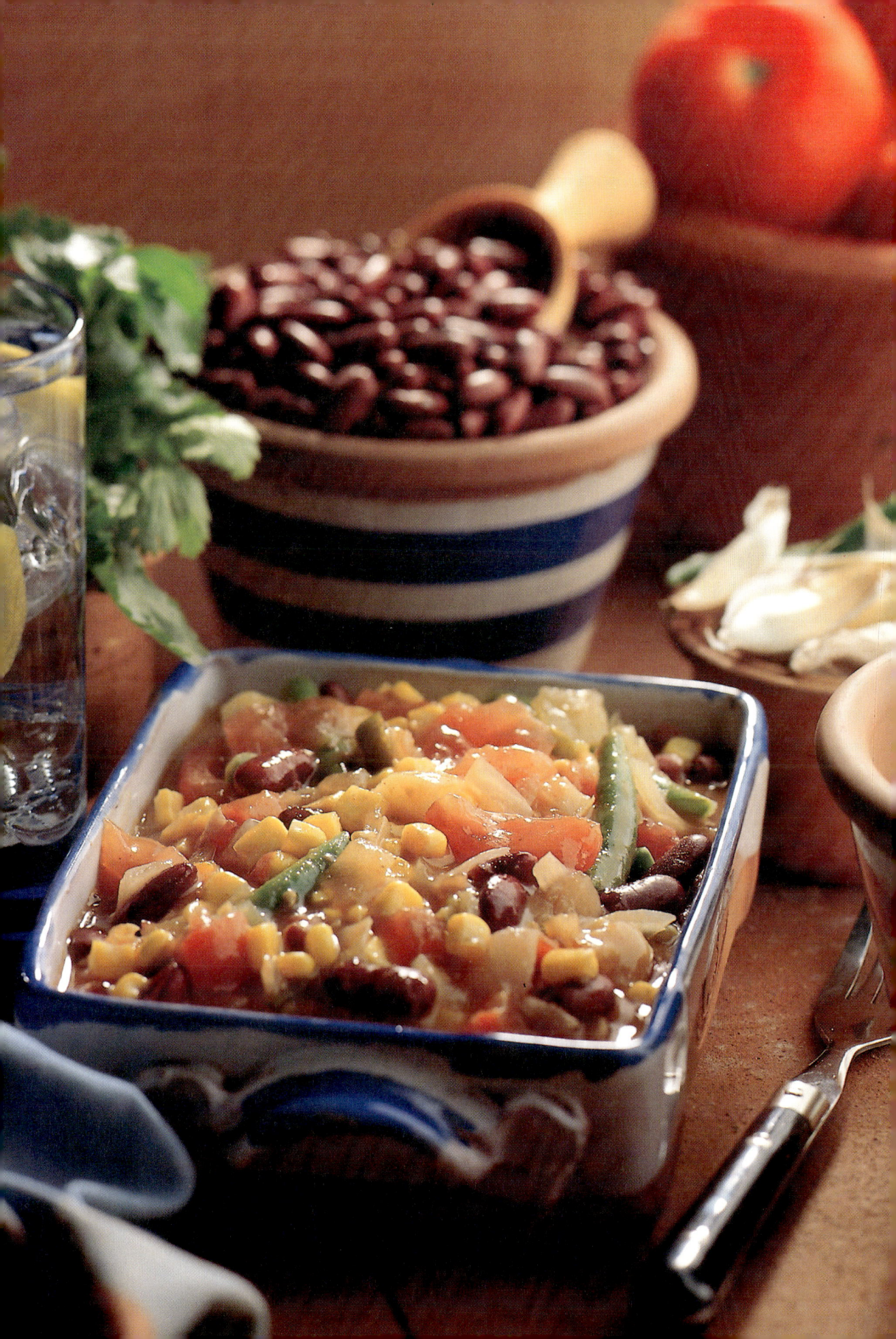

Lettuce Rolls in Lemon Sauce

1 iceberg lettuce

FILLING

160g brown rice

2 teaspoons olive oil

1/2 cup chopped onion

1/2 cup chopped fennel bulb

2 teaspoons finely grated lemon rind

80g currants

1 1/2 tablespoons chopped fresh parsley

3 tablespoons lemon juice

Freshly ground black pepper to season

LEMON SAUCE

1 cup vegetable stock

3 teaspoons plain flour

25g light cream cheese

Grated rind 1 lemon

1. To prepare the filling, cook the rice in boiling water for 35 minutes or until tender. Drain, rinse and shake well to dry. Measure to ensure you have 4 cups.

2. Heat the oil in a frying pan and cook the onion and fennel until soft but not brown.

3. Stir in the cooked rice, lemon rind, currants, parsley, lemon juice and pepper.

4. Carefully separate 12 lettuce leaves and cut out the stalk from the core end. Blanch 6 leaves at a time in boiling water for 1 minute, drain well and dry each leaf on absorbent paper.

5. Divide the filling into 12 equal portions and wrap each portion in a blanched lettuce leaf.

6. Arrange the lettuce rolls in a single layer in a microwave-safe or ovenproof dish.

7. To prepare the sauce, blend the stock, flour, cream cheese and lemon rind. Cook in a saucepan or in the microwave on 100% power for 2 to 3 minutes or until the sauce thickens.

8. Pour the sauce over the lettuce rolls and cover. Cook in the microwave on 100% power for 7 minutes. Leave to stand for 1 minute before serving. Alternatively cover and cook in the oven at 180°C for 30 minutes until hot. Serve three rolls each.

NOTE: Remember to serve some protein with this recipe.

Variation

▶ You can also make this recipe using cabbage or spinach but lettuce is softer. Parboiled wholemeal rice cuts the cooking time of the rice by half.

Cook's Tip

▶ If you buy the fennel bulbs as small as possible, they will have a sweeter taste which will complement the subtle flavour of the lettuce.

SERVES 4

EACH SERVE PROVIDES:
1 Fruit, 1 1/2 Vegetable,
1/2 Fat, 2 Bread,
100 Optional Kilojoules.
PER SERVE:
5g Fat, 7g Dietary Fibre.

Golden Filo Parcels

4 teaspoons poly-unsaturated margarine

2 tablespoons skim milk

120g filo pastry

FILLING

2 cups cooked English spinach

120g ricotta cheese

1 egg

100g feta cheese, diced or crumbled

80g currants

Nutmeg to season

1. To prepare the filling, blend or process the spinach, ricotta cheese and egg until smooth. Transfer to a bowl and fold in the feta cheese, currants and nutmeg.

2. Melt the margarine in a pan with the milk.

3. Take one sheet of filo pastry and fold in half lengthways. Brush with the milk.

4. Place a spoonful of filling in the top left hand corner. Bring the top right hand corner over to meet the other side of the pastry strip, forming a triangle.

5. Continue to fold the pastry down the length of the filo sheet so you form a triangular package which completely encloses its filling. Do not fold the pastry too tightly, as the filling will expand during cooking.

6. Repeat with the remaining mixture, making 12 parcels in total.

7. Place each parcel on a wetted baking tray and brush the tops with a little milk.

8. Bake at 190°C for 20 to 25 minutes until the parcels are golden brown and crispy. Serve immediately.

Cook's Tip

▶ These parcels can be served with the pumpkin sauce featured on page 60.

SERVES 4

EACH SERVE PROVIDES:
1 Fruit, 1 Vegetable, 1 Fat,
2 Protein, 1 Bread,
15 Optional Kilojoules.
PER SERVE:
5g Fat, 2g Dietary Fibre.

Stylish Curried Eggs

4 cups cooked noodles
or pasta, hot

Fresh coriander or parsley
to garnish

SAUCE

1 teaspoon vegetable oil

1 teaspoon sesame oil

1 green chilli, seeded and
chopped

1 clove garlic, crushed

2 teaspoons chopped
fresh ginger

1 cup diced red capsicum

3/4 cup finely chopped
spring onions

2 teaspoons each ground
cumin and coriander

3 teaspoons cornflour

1 cup vegetable stock

3/4 cup natural
low-fat yoghurt

Few drops coconut
essence

2 tablespoons chopped
fresh coriander or parsley

8 hard-cooked eggs

Coriander to garnish

1 To prepare the sauce, heat the oils in a saucepan and cook the chilli, garlic, ginger, capsicum and spring onions for about 5 minutes until they are soft but not brown.

2 Stir through the cumin and coriander.

3 Mix the cornflour with the stock and stir into the vegetables. Cook over a low heat until the sauce thickens.

4 Fold in the yoghurt, coconut essence and fresh coriander.

5 Cut the hard-cooked eggs in half and fold into the sauce. Warm through gently.

6 Serve over hot noodles or pasta. Garnish with coriander before serving.

Cook's Tip

▶ Wash your hands well after using chillies as they will burn your eyes if you rub them.

SERVES 4

EACH SERVE PROVIDES:
1 Vegetable, 1/2 Fat,
2 Protein, 2 Bread,
1/4 Milk,
50 Optional Kilojoules.
PER SERVE:
15g Fat, 4g Dietary Fibre.

Stylish Curried Eggs.

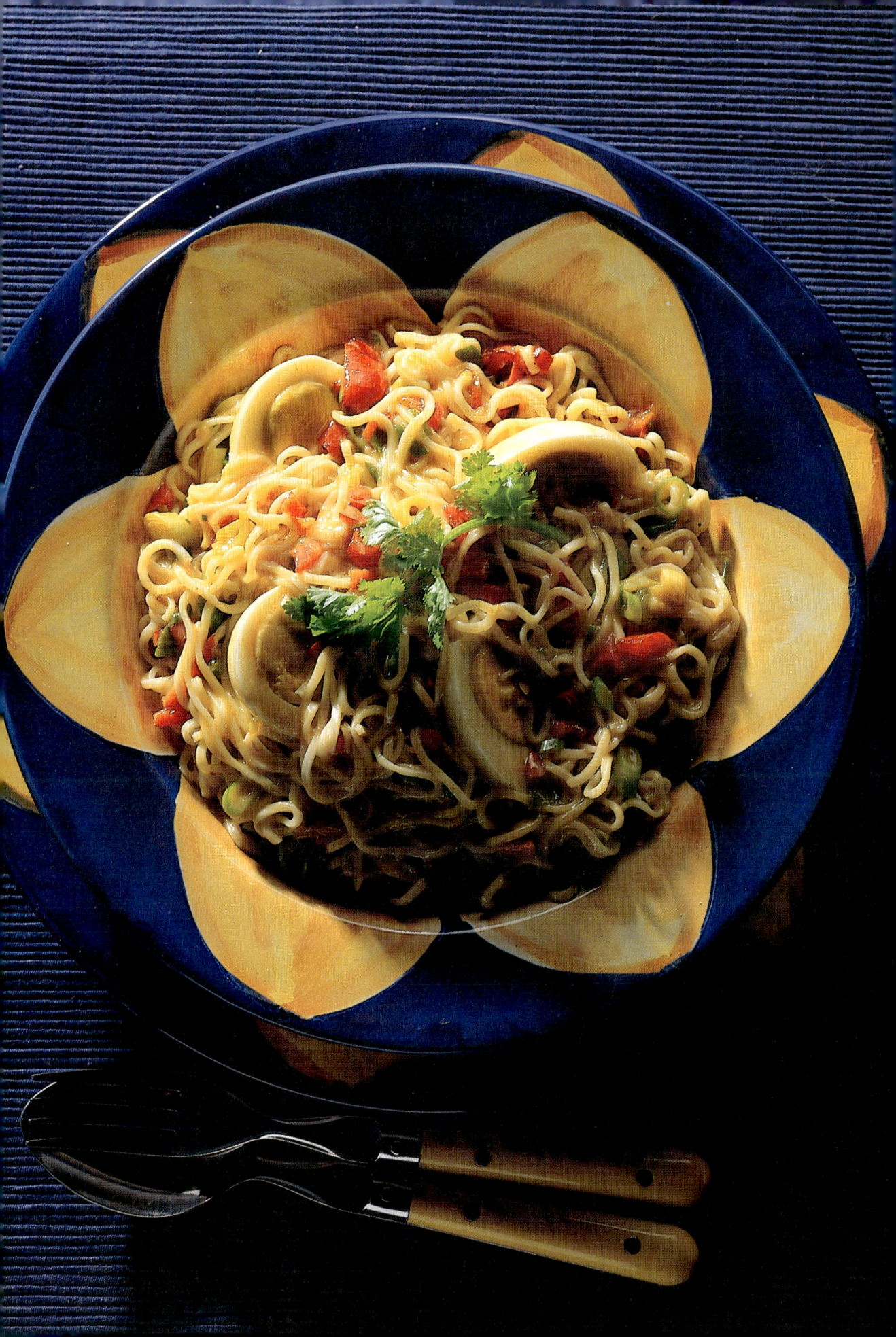

Lentils in Sweet Chilli Sauce

160g brown lentils

2 green chillies, seeded and diced

2 teaspoons chopped fresh ginger

$^1/_2$ cup finely chopped onion

1 teaspoon sesame oil

1 cup diced red capsicum

$1^1/_2$ cups diced green capsicum

$^1/_2$ cup tomato paste

3 teaspoons oyster sauce

3 teaspoons white wine vinegar

1 teaspoon cornflour

2 teaspoons honey

$^1/_4$ cup vegetable stock

2 cups sliced cucumber

2 tablespoons chopped fresh coriander to garnish

Microwave Method

1. In a saucepan, cook the lentils in boiling water for about 30 minutes until they are tender. Drain and set aside.

2. Put the chillies, ginger, onion and sesame oil in a microwave-safe bowl and cover loosely. Cook on 100% power for 4 minutes. Add the capsicum and tomato paste, and cook on 100% power for 2 minutes.

3. In a jug or bowl, combine the oyster sauce, wine vinegar, cornflour, honey and stock. Stir to dissolve the cornflour. Stir into the hot chilli mixture. Cook on 100% power for 1 minute.

4. Add the drained lentils and cucumber, mixing well. Cook on 70% power for 3 to 4 minutes until the lentils are very hot. Serve garnished with fresh coriander.

Variation

▶ Use other pulses in place of lentils. Pinto beans or baby lima beans taste good. They need to soak for about 8 hours before cooking.

Cook's Tip

▶ Accompany with steamed vegetables, including pumpkin, which goes well with all these flavours.

SERVES 4

EACH SERVE PROVIDES:
3 Vegetable, $^1/_4$ Fat,
2 Protein,
105 Optional Kilojoules.
PER SERVE:
2g Fat, $6^1/_2$g Dietary Fibre.

Vegetable Pot Au Feu

2 cups vegetable stock

1 cup sliced green beans

2 cups whole baby carrots, scrubbed

2 cups fresh or frozen broad beans

2 teaspoons olive oil

$^1/_2$ cup chopped onion

$^1/_2$ cup sliced celery

1 cup chopped red capsicum

$1^1/_2$ tablespoons plain flour

125 mL dry white wine

$1^1/_2$ cups sliced zucchini

6 sun-dried tomato halves (not packed in oil)

2 tablespoons chopped fresh oregano

25g light sour cream

Freshly ground black pepper to season

1. Heat the stock and blanch the green beans for 3 to 4 minutes. Drain, reserving the stock.

2. Cook the whole carrots in the reserved stock for 4 to 5 minutes. Drain, again reserving the stock.

3. Cook the broad beans in the reserved stock for 2 to 3 minutes and drain, reserving the stock. Boil the remaining stock until it reduces to $1^1/_2$ cups and then set aside. Peel the broad beans.

4. Heat the oil in a frying pan and gently cook the onion and celery for 4 to 5 minutes until soft but not brown. Add the capsicum and cook until just tender.

5. Stir in the flour. Cook for 2 to 3 minutes until frothy, stirring continuously. Gradually add the wine and reduced stock, stirring constantly. Cook until the sauce begins to thicken slightly.

6. Add the carrots, green beans, zucchini, tomato halves and oregano. Cover and simmer very gently for 10 to 12 minutes or until the vegetables are tender.

7. Add the peeled broad beans, sour cream and pepper. Serve immediately.

NOTE: Remember to serve some protein with this recipe.

Cook's Tip

▶ Broad beans are best peeled, as the centre of the bean is very different from the tough outer skins.

SERVES 4

EACH SERVE PROVIDES:
5 Vegetable, $^1/_2$ Fat,
140 Optional Kilojoules.
PER SERVE:
$4^1/_2$g Fat, 11g Dietary Fibre.

Pasta with Brie and Green Beans

3 cups frozen green beans

1 teaspoon olive oil

2 cloves garlic, crushed

$1/2$ cup chopped spring onions

$1^{1}/_{2}$ cups vegetable stock

$1^{1}/_{2}$ tablespoons plain flour

120g soft blue Brie style cheese, thinly sliced

Pepper to season

4 cups cooked pasta of your choice, hot

1. Blanch the beans in boiling water until almost cooked and drain well.

2. Heat the oil in a frying pan, and cook the garlic and spring onions over a moderate heat for about 3 minutes.

3. Add $1^{1}/_{4}$ cups of the stock and simmer for 3 to 5 minutes. Blend the flour with the remaining stock, mix into the sauce and cook over a low heat until the sauce thickens.

4. Add the blue cheese and beans, and toss only until the cheese begins to melt. Season well with pepper.

5. Toss the sauce through freshly cooked pasta and serve hot.

Microwave Method

1. Blanch the beans in the microwave until almost cooked. Set aside.

2. Put the oil, garlic and spring onions in a microwave-safe dish. Cover and cook on 100% power for $1^{1}/_{2}$ minutes.

3. Blend the stock and flour and add to the dish with the beans. Cover and cook on 100% power for $3^{1}/_{2}$ to $4^{1}/_{2}$ minutes until the sauce thickens, stirring 2 to 3 times during the cooking time.

4. Stir in the cheese and season with pepper. Toss the sauce through freshly cooked pasta and serve hot.

SERVES 4

EACH SERVE PROVIDES:
$1^{3}/_{4}$ Vegetable, $1/4$ Fat,
$1^{1}/_{2}$ Protein, 2 Bread,
95 Optional Kilojoules.
PER SERVE:
11g Fat, 6g Dietary Fibre.

Pasta with Brie and Green Beans.

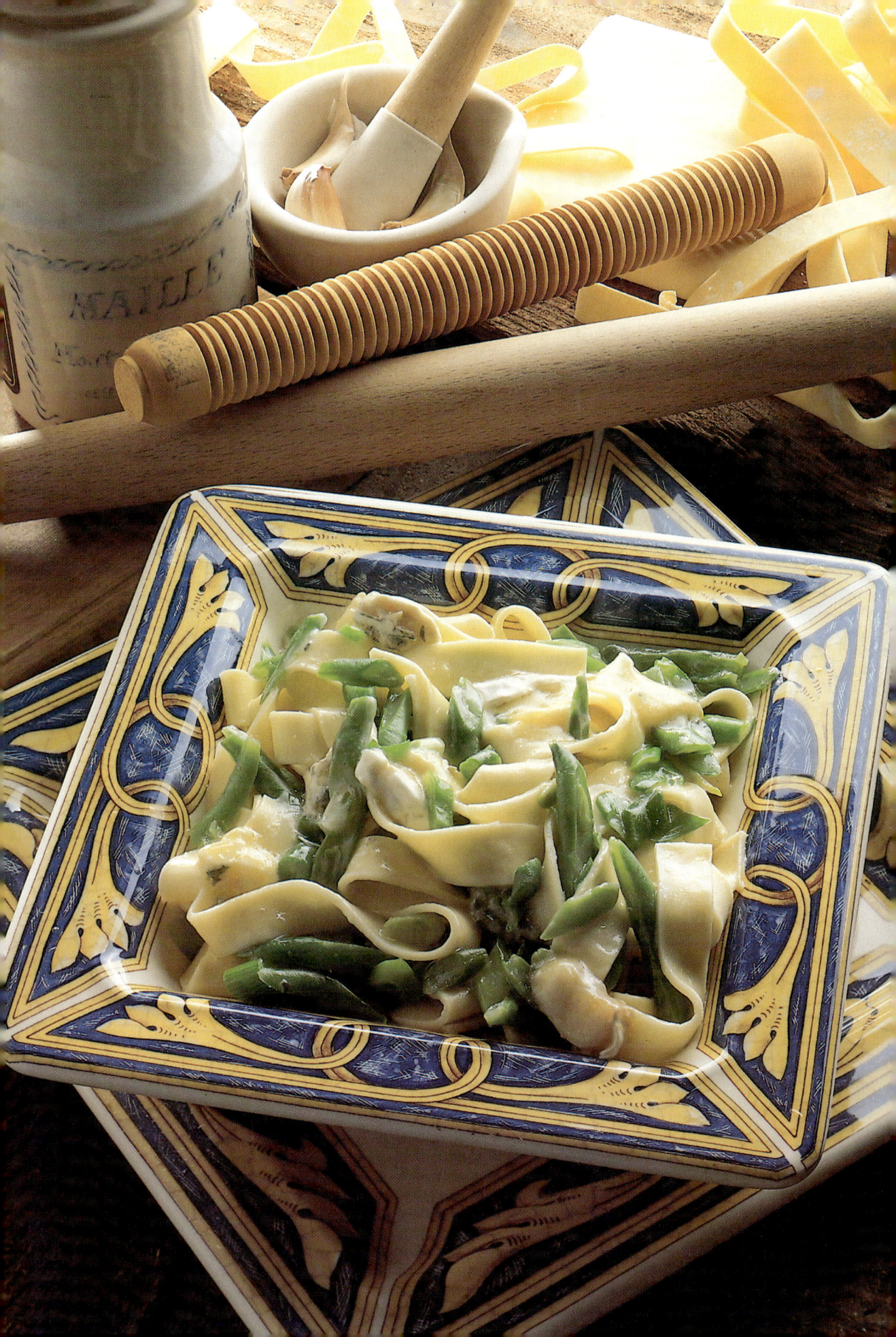

Tofu and Mushroom Stir-fry

400g tofu, diced

1 clove garlic, crushed

1 teaspoon minced fresh ginger

1 tablespoon Indonesian soy sauce (kepjap manis)

60mL dry sherry

1 teaspoon vegetable stock powder

2 cups broccoli florets

3 teaspoons vegetable oil

1 cup sliced leeks

3 cups sliced mushrooms

1¼ cups water

3 teaspoons cornflour

½ teaspoon cracked black pepper

1 teaspoon sesame oil

1. In a bowl, toss the tofu, garlic, ginger, soy sauce, sherry and vegetable stock powder. Set aside for 10 minutes.

2. Blanch the broccoli quickly, either in boiling water or in the microwave.

3. Heat the oil in a frying pan and cook the leeks and mushrooms, tossing briefly for about 5 minutes.

4. Stir in the tofu mixture and broccoli.

5. Mix the water and cornflour, and pour into the pan. Cook until the sauce thickens. Season with the pepper and sesame oil.

Variation

▶ While this is a vegetarian option, tofu can be omitted and meat or poultry used. Beef or chicken would be best.

Cook's Tip

▶ Serve with steamed long-grain rice.

SERVES 4

EACH SERVE PROVIDES:
3 Vegetable, 1 Fat,
1 Protein,
100 Optional Kilojoules.
PER SERVE:
9½g Fat, 6g Dietary Fibre

Summer Couscous

160g couscous

1¼ cups vegetable stock

½ cup boiling water

6 sun-dried tomato halves (not packed in oil)

4 teaspoons olive oil

1 teaspoon each finely chopped garlic and fresh ginger

2 teaspoons cumin

¼ cup tomato paste

1 cup whole baby carrots

1 cup baby sweet corn

1 cup sliced zucchini

1 cup whole baby leeks or spring onions, trimmed

2 cups sliced asparagus

1 cup diced eggplant

1½ cups vegetable stock, hot

½ cup natural low-fat yoghurt

Chopped fresh mint to garnish

1. Put the couscous and 1¼ cups stock in a bowl, cover and leave for 30 minutes.

2. Pour ½ cup boiling water over the sun-dried tomatoes and leave for 5 minutes. Drain, reserving the liquid, and cut the tomatoes into thin strips.

3. Heat the oil in a large saucepan and cook the garlic, ginger and cumin for 1 to 2 minutes. Add the tomato paste and cook for 1 to 2 minutes, stirring often until the paste darkens a little.

4. Add the sun-dried tomatoes, reserved liquid, carrots, corn, zucchini, leeks, asparagus, eggplant and 1½ cups stock. Simmer for about 10 minutes until the vegetables are just cooked but not overdone.

5. Reheat the couscous for 2 minutes on top of the stove over low heat or alternatively, in the microwave. Serve the couscous in bowls and pour over equal amounts of the vegetable mixture. Garnish with yoghurt and mint.

Variation

▶ If you would like the sauce on the couscous to be a little thicker, add 2 teaspoons cornflour after the sauce has simmered for about 8 minutes. Add 25 Optional Kilojoules per serve.

SERVES 4

EACH SERVE PROVIDES:
4 Vegetable, 1 Fat,
2½ Bread, ¼ Milk,
40 Optional Kilojoules.
PER SERVE:
7g Fat, 11g Dietary Fibre.

Burghul Salad

120g burghul wheat

1¼ cups boiling water

¼ teaspoon salt

160g feta cheese

2 cups sliced apricots

2 cups diced cucumber

2 tablespoons chopped
fresh mint

40g stoned black olives

Bitter lettuce
(e.g. witloof, raddichio
and curly endive)
leaves to serve

DRESSING

2 tablespoons white wine
vinegar

2 teaspoons wholegrain
mustard

1 teaspoon honey

1. Put the burghul wheat into a bowl. Bring the water and salt to the boil. Pour over the burghul and leave for 30 minutes. Drain away any water that may remain and dry the wheat if you wish, on absorbent paper.

2. In a large bowl, combine the burghul, feta, apricots, cucumber, mint and olives.

3. In a small bowl, mix all the dressing ingredients. Toss dressing through the salad. Serve with lettuce.

Variation

▶ In place of burghul, use cooked rice or couscous.

Cook's Tip

▶ Salted water is called for in this recipe as the burghul needs it for flavour. You can use vegetable stock instead, but remember to add the extra Optional Kilojoules.

SERVES 4

EACH SERVE PROVIDES:
1 Fruit, 1 Vegetable,
2 Protein, 1½ Bread,
40 Optional Kilojoules.
PER SERVE:
11g Fat, 6½g Dietary Fibre.

Burghul Salad.

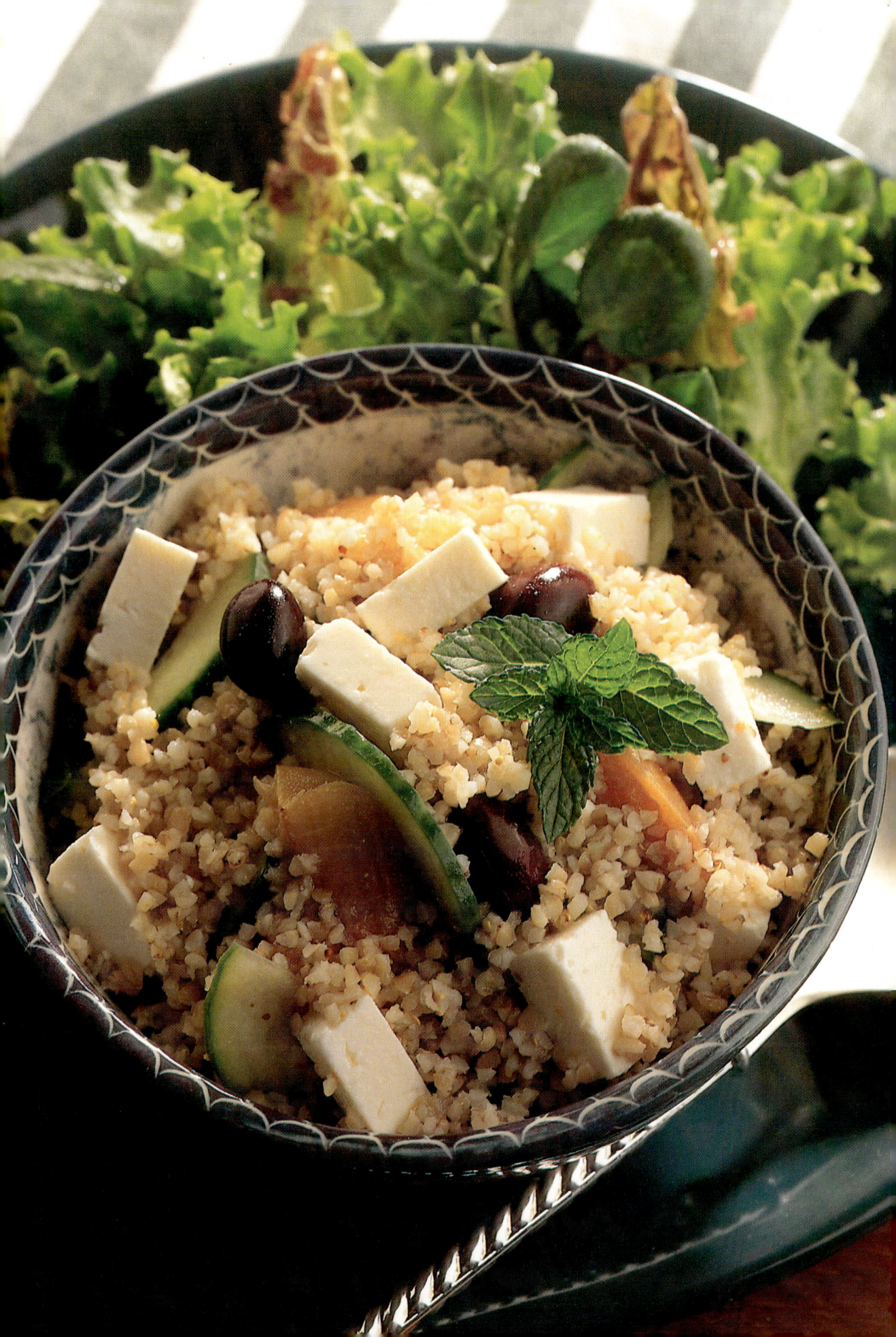

Italian Pie

BASE

1 cup cooked English spinach, roughly chopped

180g ricotta cheese

1 egg

Pinch pepper and nutmeg

FILLING

2 teaspoons olive oil

2 cups diced eggplant

1 cup diced red capsicum

1/2 cup finely diced fennel bulb

3 cloves garlic, crushed

1/2 cup chopped spring onions

1/4 cup chopped fresh basil, fennel fronds or dill

1 cup tomato purée

TOPPING

2 slices wholemeal bread

2 teaspoons poly-unsaturated margarine

1. To prepare the base, blend or process the spinach, ricotta cheese and egg, seasoning well with pepper and nutmeg. Press evenly over the base of a 4-cup capacity ovenproof pie dish.

2. To prepare the filling, heat the oil in a frying pan and cook the eggplant, capsicum, fennel, garlic and spring onions, over a moderate heat for about 5 minutes until lightly browned. Stir in the basil and tomato purée.

3. Spread the filling over the base.

4. To prepare the topping, process the bread to crumbs with the margarine and sprinkle over the top of the pie.

5. Bake at 180°C for about 40 to 45 minutes until golden. Serve with slices of fresh tomato if desired.

Variations

▶ You can use cottage cheese instead of ricotta but it would be best to sieve it first.

▶ Use silverbeet if you do not have spinach. Tear the leaves from the coarse white stem, chop the white part finely and add to the filling.

▶ If you do not have a fennel bulb, use another vegetable such as capsicum or zucchini.

SERVES 4

EACH SERVE PROVIDES:
3 Vegetable, 1 Fat,
1 Protein, 1/2 Bread.
PER SERVE:
12g Fat, 8g Dietary Fibre.

Lentil and Mushroom Loaf

160g brown lentils

2 cups vegetable stock

4 teaspoons olive oil

1 clove garlic, crushed

1½ cups finely chopped leeks

3 cups finely chopped mushrooms

3 eggs

50g light sour cream

1 teaspoon paprika

1 tablespoon chopped fresh parsley

100g grated sweet potatoes

Pepper to season

1. Simmer the lentils in the stock for about 30 minutes until they are tender. Drain and set aside.

2. Heat the oil in a frying pan and cook the garlic and leeks over a moderate heat for about 5 minutes until they are soft but not brown. Add the mushrooms and cook for about 5 minutes.

3. In a bowl, beat together the eggs and sour cream. Stir in the cooked lentils, cooked vegetables, paprika, parsley and sweet potatoes. Season well with pepper.

4. Line a 4-cup capacity loaf tin with baking paper and pour in the mixture. Cover with foil. Bake at 180°C for 45 to 50 minutes or until the loaf has set. Leave for 10 minutes before slicing. Serve hot or warm.

Microwave Method

1. Follow the recipe steps 1, 2, and 3.

2. Line a microwave-safe 4-cup capacity loaf tin with non-stick baking paper. Pour in the mixture. Cover loosely with baking paper. Cook on 70% power for 10 minutes. Leave for 5 minutes. The loaf should be firm to the touch.

Cook's Tip

▶ Use a sharply serrated knife to cut the lentil loaf cleanly.

SERVES 4

EACH SERVE PROVIDES:
2¼ Vegetable, 1 Fat,
2¾ Protein, ¼ Bread,
125 Optional Kilojoules.
PER SERVE:
13g Fat, 9g Dietary Fibre.

SWEET TREATS

Sweets are almost everyone's favourite course and probably the area where we fall down the most with the kilojoules when we are cooking. These low-energy desserts are delicious and look stunning when presented. Most of these scrumptious ideas are based on fruit, which should become one of your best friends. Fruit will also help cleanse the palate after dinner. These recipes will help revitalise your thoughts about fruit desserts, the perfect way to end a meal.

Fruit Shortcakes

160g plain flour

1 teaspoon
baking powder

$^1/_2$ teaspoon baking soda
(bicarbonate of soda)

3 teaspoons castor sugar

40g polyunsaturated
margarine

$^1/_2$ cup buttermilk

2 cups fresh berries

$^1/_2$ cup natural low-fat
yoghurt (fruit or plain)

2 cups pawpaw, puréed

1. Sift the flour, baking powder, baking soda and sugar into a bowl. Rub in the margarine with your fingertips. Stir in the buttermilk until the mixture forms a soft dough.

2. Turn the dough onto a lightly floured board and roll flat until it is 1cm thick. Fold in half and roll out again.

3. Cut out eight small rounds and place on a wetted tray. Bake at 220°C for 15 minutes until well risen and golden.

4. Cool on a wire rack. Split in half (they will split where they were folded). Fill with equal amounts of fresh berries and yoghurt.

5. Place two cakes on each plate with one quarter of the pawpaw purée.

SERVES 4

WITH 2 CAKES PER PERSON.
EACH SERVE PROVIDES:
1 Fruit, 2 Fat, 2 Bread, $^1/_4$ Milk,
140 Optional Kilojoules.
PER SERVE:
$9^1/_2$g Fat, 5g Dietary Fibre.

Fruit Shortcakes.

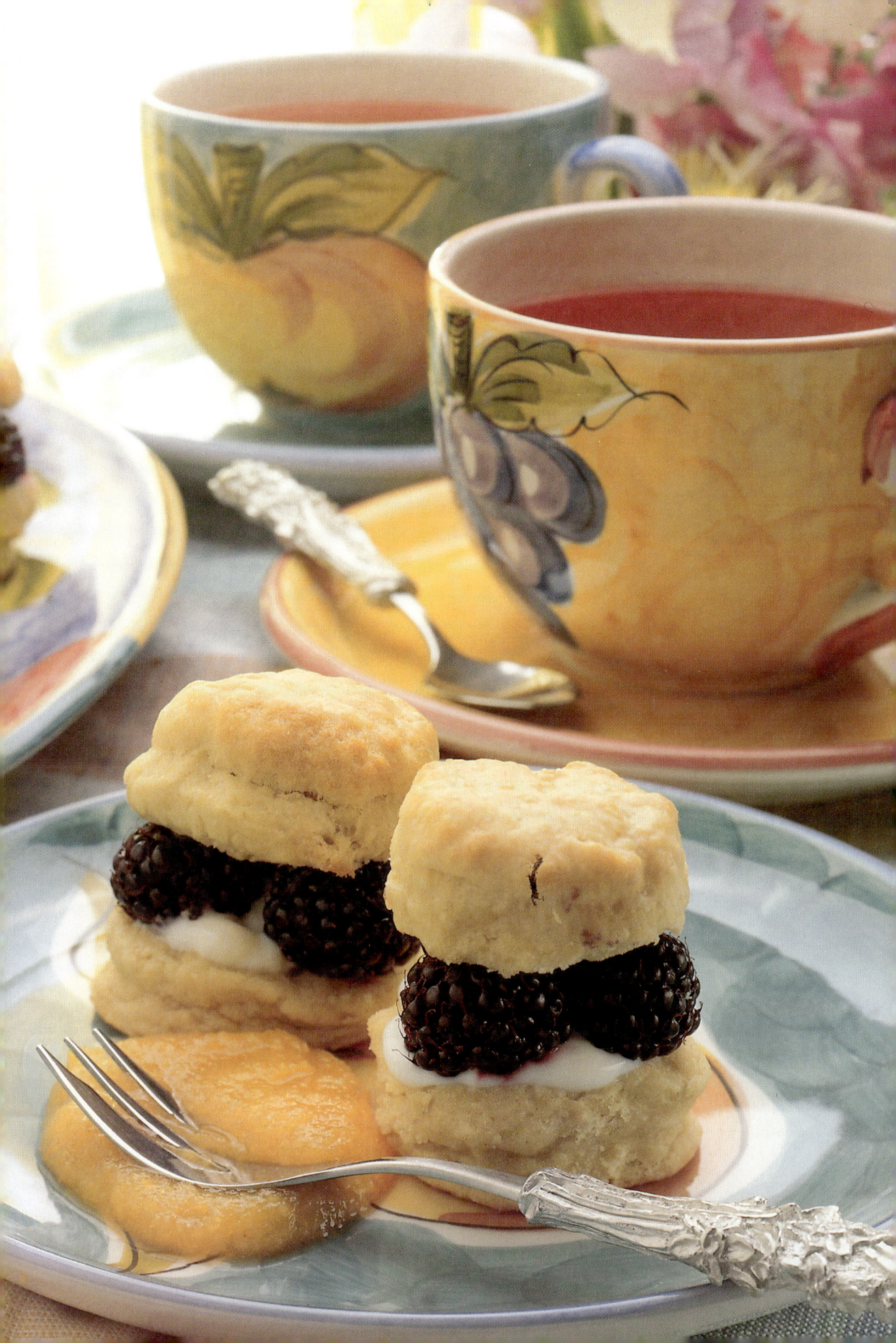

Blueberry Cobbler

4 apples

1½ cups blueberries

½ cup fresh orange juice

COBBLER
TOPPING

120g plain flour

1¾ teaspoons baking
powder

½ teaspoon cinnamon

3 teaspoons castor sugar

Grated rind 1 orange

1 egg, beaten

¼ cup skim milk

1. Peel, core and slice the apples. Place them in a deep dish with the blueberries and orange juice and mix through.

2. To prepare the topping, sift the flour, baking powder, cinnamon and castor sugar into a bowl. Stir in the orange rind. Mix in the beaten egg and sufficient milk to form a soft dough.

3. Turn out onto a lightly floured board and knead together. Roll out to about 1cm thick. Cut into 4cm rounds and arrange on top of the berries, around the edge of the dish.

4. Bake at 190°C for 20 minutes or until the cobbler is well risen and golden, and the apples are soft and cooked. Serve hot or warm.

Variations

▶ Use different fruits, such as pears and apricots, or apples and raspberries.

▶ Keep frozen fruits on hand, especially the summer berries, as they will add variety throughout the winter months.

SERVES 4

EACH SERVE PROVIDES:
2 Fruit, ¼ Protein,
1½ Bread,
90 Optional Kilojoules.
PER SERVE:
2g Fat, 5½g Dietary Fibre.

Fruit with Ginger Custard

2 cups skim milk

1 teaspoon honey

$^1/_4$ teaspoon ground ginger

2 tablespoons cornflour

3 cups sliced or diced mixed seasonal fruit

$1^1/_2$ tablespoons castor sugar

1. Heat $1^3/_4$ cups milk to scalding point. Blend the remaining milk with the honey, ginger and cornflour. Stir into the hot milk. Cook until the mixture thickens.

2. Arrange the fruit in a shallow ovenproof dish and spoon over the warm custard. Sprinkle the castor sugar on top.

3. Heat the grill. Grill the custard until the sugar caramelises and turns golden. Take care not to burn the sugar. Serve hot or warm.

Cook's Tip

▶ The fruit can be berry, stone or pip fruit. It tastes better if the stone and pip fruit are slightly cooked first. Poach them in a little water or cook them in the microwave.

SERVES 4

EACH SERVE PROVIDES:
$1^1/_2$ Fruit, $^1/_2$ Milk,
185 Optional Kilojoules.
PER SERVE:
$^1/_2$g Fat, 3g Dietary Fibre.

Strawberries in Wine Jelly

1 cup water

2 tablespoons lemon juice

60mL sweet wine

Peeled rind $\frac{1}{2}$ lemon

2 teaspoons gelatine

2 tablespoons water

2 cups sliced strawberries

Fresh herb flowers to garnish (optional)

1. In a saucepan, heat 1 cup water, lemon juice, wine and lemon rind, and bring to the boil. Simmer for 5 minutes.

2. Sprinkle the gelatine over 2 tablespoons water and leave to swell. Dissolve over hot water or place in the microwave on 100% power for 10 to 15 seconds.

3. Blend the gelatine into the lemon mixture. Stir well and remove from the heat. Leave to cool until almost set.

4. Put the strawberries in four $\frac{3}{4}$-cup capacity moulds and pour the lemon mixture over the strawberries. Chill in the refrigerator for at least 4 hours until well set.

5. Remove from the refrigerator 30 minutes before serving to bring the jelly to room temperature. This will bring out a stronger flavour.

SERVES 4

EACH SERVE PROVIDES:
$\frac{1}{2}$ Fruit,
100 Optional Kilojoules.
PER SERVE:
0g Fat, 2g Dietary Fibre.

Strawberries in Wine Jelly (front);
Jaffaberry Sherbet (page 100).

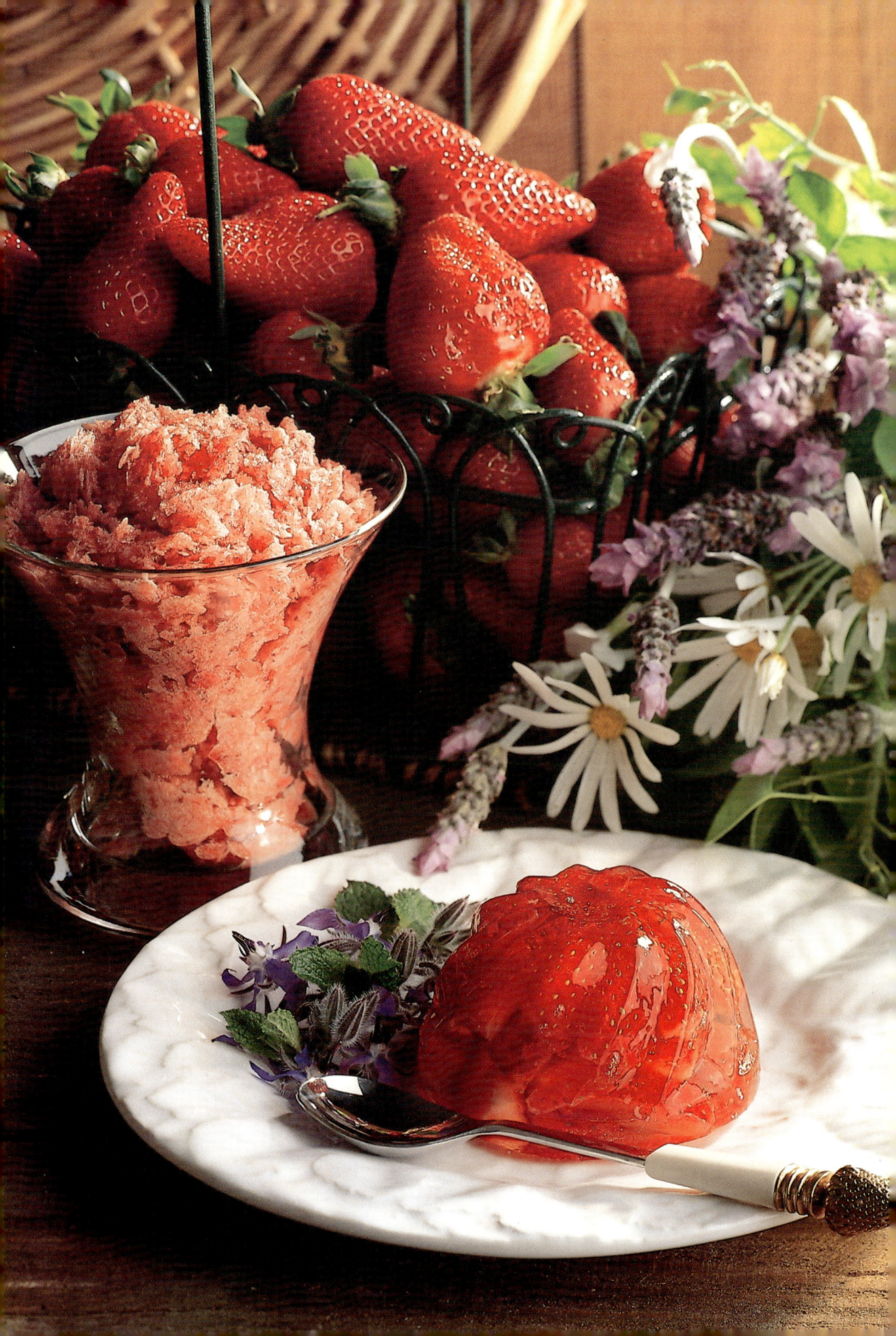

Jaffaberry Sherbet

2 cups finely sliced rhubarb

2 teaspoons grated orange rind

$1/2$ cup orange juice

2 cups fresh or frozen strawberries

3 egg whites

$1^1/2$ tablespoons castor sugar

1. Simmer the rhubarb, orange rind and half the orange juice in a saucepan for 4 to 5 minutes until the rhubarb begins to soften.

2. Hull and halve the strawberries and add to the pan. Simmer for a further 5 minutes. Mash the fruits with a fork. Stir in the remaining orange juice.

3. Leave to cool. Turn into a freezer tray and freeze until slightly mushy. Break up the fruit mixture with a fork to form small ice particles.

4. In a clean glass bowl, beat the egg whites with the sugar until glossy and thick. Fold into the fruit mixture. Freeze until firm.

5. Remove from the freezer 20 minutes before serving or place in the microwave for 1 minute on defrost setting. Scoop equal quantities into six dishes.

SERVES 6

EACH SERVE PROVIDES:
$3/4$ Fruit, $1/2$ Vegetable,
145 Optional Kilojoules.
PER SERVE:
0g Fat, $2^1/2$g Dietary Fibre.

Mulled Pears

125mL red wine

¹/₄ cup water

¹/₂ cup orange juice

Strip lemon rind

1 cinnamon stick

2 whole cloves

4 pears

120g ricotta cheese

1. In a saucepan, simmer the red wine, water, orange juice, lemon rind, cinnamon stick and cloves for about 5 minutes over a low heat.

2. Peel, core and halve the pears. Gently simmer them in the mulled wine for about 10 minutes, turning once if necessary. The pears should be cooked, giving little resistance when tested with a skewer.

3. Cool the pears in the wine so they develop a stronger flavour. Remove the spices and the lemon rind.

4. Reheat the pears if you want to serve them hot. Serve cut side uppermost, filled with ricotta cheese.

Variation

▶ Use apples or nashi fruit in place of pears.

SERVES 4

EACH SERVE PROVIDES:
1¹/₄ Fruit, ¹/₂ Protein,
100 Optional Kilojoules.
PER SERVE:
3¹/₂g Fat, 4g Dietary Fibre.

Apple and Ginger Mousse

4 small apples

1 teaspoon ground ginger

$^{1}/_{4}$ cup water

3 teaspoons gelatine

2 egg whites

1 tablespoon sugar

150g natural
low-fat yoghurt

Grated rind 1 lemon

$^{1}/_{2}$ apple, sliced and
lemon rind to garnish

1. Peel, core and slice the apples. Cook them in a saucepan with the ginger and 1 tablespoon water until soft and mushy. Alternatively, place apples, ginger and water in a microwave-safe bowl, cover and cook on 100% power for 8 minutes.

2. Blend or process the apples until very smooth.

3. Sprinkle the gelatine over the remaining water and leave to swell. Dissolve over hot water or place in the microwave on 100% power for 10 to 15 seconds. Mix into the apple purée. Set aside until the mixture cools and thickens.

4. Whisk the egg whites in a clean bowl until they form soft peaks. Beat in the sugar until the mixture resembles meringue.

5. Fold the yoghurt, lemon rind and egg whites into the cooled apple purée. Turn into a wetted loaf tin and refrigerate for 4 hours until the mousse has set.

6. Turn out onto a platter. Serve sliced, garnished with apple slices and lemon rind.

Variations

▶ You can also make this mousse with pears or peaches.

▶ Use artificial sweetener to replace the sugar and reduce the Optional Kilojoules per serving by 50.

Cook's Tip

▶ Choose good flavoured apples for this dessert.

A Note On Turning Out Moulded Foods

▶ Fill the sink with warm water. Take your mould and dip it quickly up to the rim and then take it straight out of the water. Invert the mould onto a platter, give it a few firm shakes and the mould should release. If it doesn't, then repeat the process. The thicker the mould, the longer it will take to cool. Cake tin style moulds are easier to turn food out of. Crockery moulds are best avoided.

SERVES 8

EACH SERVE PROVIDES:
$^{1}/_{2}$ Fruit, $^{1}/_{4}$ Milk,
70 Optional Kilojoules.
PER SERVE:
0g Fat, $1^{1}/_{2}$g Dietary Fibre.

Apple and Ginger Mousse (on plate);
Pina Colada Mousse (page 104).

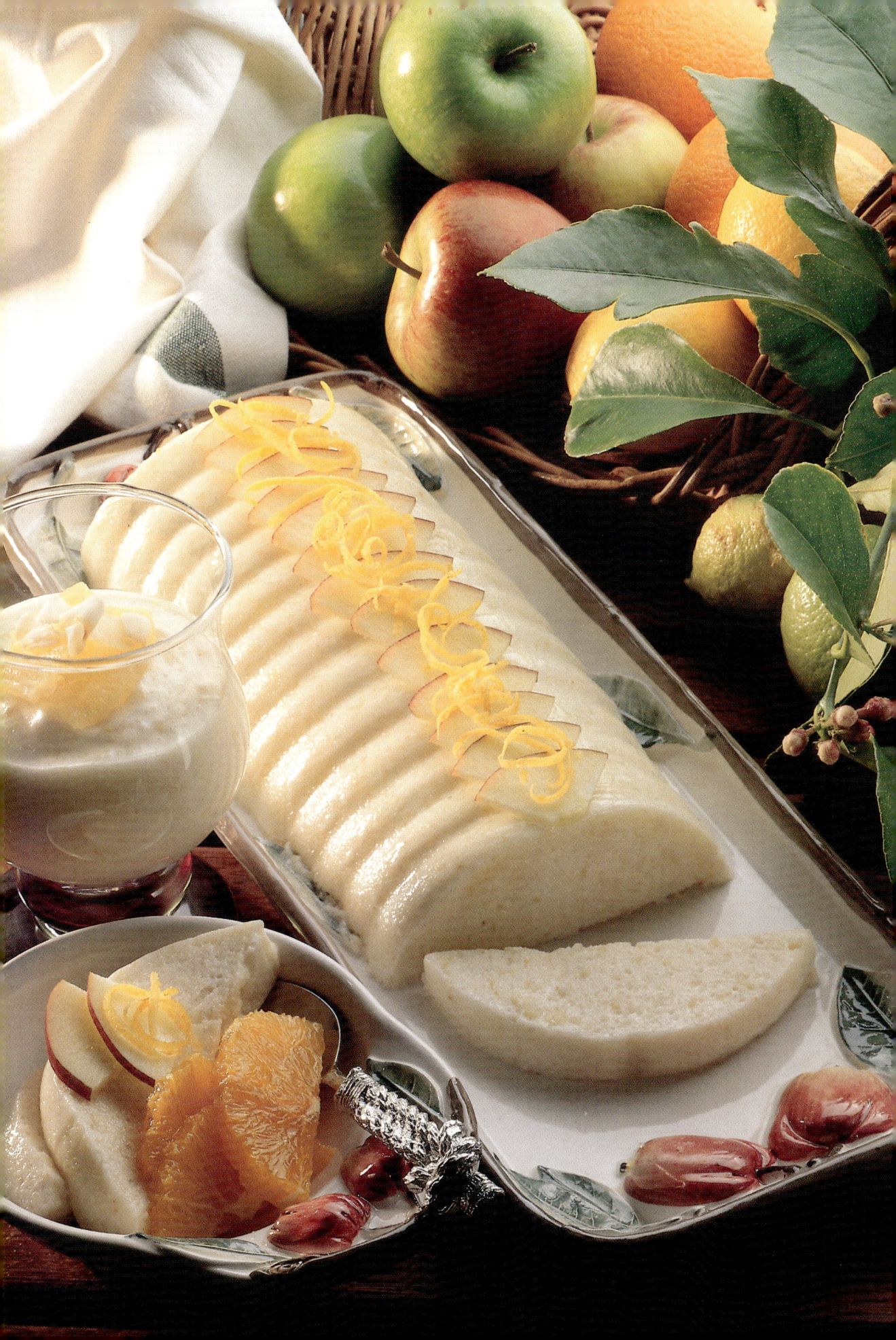

Pina Colada Mousse

2 cups canned crushed unsweetened pineapple in juice (see Cook's Tip)

3 teaspoons gelatine

1 cup natural low-fat yoghurt

$1/4$ teaspoon coconut essence

2 egg whites

3 teaspoons castor sugar

2 teaspoons shredded coconut, toasted until golden

1 cup sliced pineapple

1. Strain the pineapple, reserving any juice. Mix $1/4$ cup juice with the gelatine and leave to swell. Dissolve over hot water or place in the microwave on 100% power for about 15 seconds.

2. Mix the remaining juice with the pineapple, yoghurt and coconut essence. Stir in the dissolved gelatine and set aside until the mixture thickens slightly.

3. In a clean bowl, whisk the egg whites until they are stiff but not dry. Beat in the sugar until the mixture resembles meringue.

4. Carefully fold the egg whites into the pineapple mixture and turn into a 4-cup capacity serving dish or four individual 1-cup serving dishes.

5. Chill in the refrigerator until set. Garnish with the shredded coconut and sliced pineapple.

Cook's Tip

▶ Canned pineapple must be used for this recipe, as fresh pineapple will not set with the gelatine.

SERVES 4

EACH SERVE PROVIDES:
$1^1/2$ Fruit, $1/2$ Milk,
130 Optional Kilojoules.
PER SERVE:
$1/2$g Fat, 2g Dietary Fibre.

Pictured in glass page 103.

Creme Caramels

4 cups skim milk

2 teaspoons vanilla
or lemon essence

4 eggs, well beaten

2 tablespoons
castor sugar

1 tablespoon golden syrup

2 cups sliced fresh
fruit such as apricots
or peaches

1. In a bowl beat together the milk, essence, eggs and castor sugar. Pour the mixture through a strainer to remove any egg parts.

2. Pour equal quantities into four 1-cup capacity ovenproof moulds and place in a water bath (see Cook's Tip).

3. Cook in a 180°C oven for 45 to 60 minutes or until a knife inserted into the custard comes out clean.

4. Allow the custards to cool for at least 2 hours. Run a knife around the inside of the moulds to release the custards and invert onto a serving platter.

5. Spoon 1 teaspoon of the syrup onto the top of each mould. Serve each creme caramel with ½ cup sliced fresh fruit.

Variation

▶ Use artificial sweetener instead of the castor sugar and reduce the Optional Kilojoules per serving to 100.

Cook's Tip

▶ Make a water bath by placing the casserole or pie dish in a larger pan, such as a roasting dish, transfer to the oven then pour water into the larger pan until it comes halfway up the side of the smaller dish.

SERVES 4

EACH SERVE PROVIDES:
1 Fruit, 1 Protein, 1 Milk,
215 Optional Kilojoules.
PER SERVE:
6½g Fat, 1½g Dietary Fibre.

Raspberry Cheesecake

BASE

80g plain flour

$^1/_2$ teaspoon baking powder

40g polyunsaturated margarine

Chilled water

FILLING

1 tablespoon gelatine

$^1/_4$ cup water

100g light cream cheese

600g red fruit natural low-fat yoghurt e.g. berry or plum

2 egg whites

$1^1/_2$ tablespoons castor sugar

2 cups fresh raspberries

1. To prepare the base, sift the flour and baking powder into a bowl. Rub in the margarine until the mixture resembles crumbs. Stir in enough cold water to make a stiff dough.

2. Turn the dough onto a lightly floured board and roll into a circle about 22cm wide. Place on a wetted baking tray. Prick all over with a fork.

3. Bake at 200°C for 12 to 15 minutes. While warm, cut the pastry into a 20cm circle and place in the bottom of a 20cm loose bottomed cake tin. Leave to cool.

4. To prepare the filling, sprinkle the gelatine over the water and leave to swell. Dissolve over hot water or place in the microwave on 100% power for 10 seconds.

5. Blend the softened cream cheese and yoghurt. Stir in the dissolved gelatine.

6. Whisk the egg whites in a clean bowl until they form soft peaks. Beat in the sugar until the mixture resembles meringue. Fold into the yoghurt mixture with $1^1/_2$ cups of the raspberries.

7. Turn the mixture into the prepared cake tin. Mash about half the remaining berries and drizzle over the top. Drop the remaining whole berries on top so that they sink. Refrigerate for at least 4 hours until set. Serve sliced.

SERVES 8

EACH SERVE PROVIDES:
$^1/_4$ Fruit, 1 Fat,
$^1/_2$ Bread, $^1/_2$ Milk,
200 Optional Kilojoules.
PER SERVE:
$6^1/_2$g Fat, 3g Dietary Fibre.

Raspberry Cheesecake.

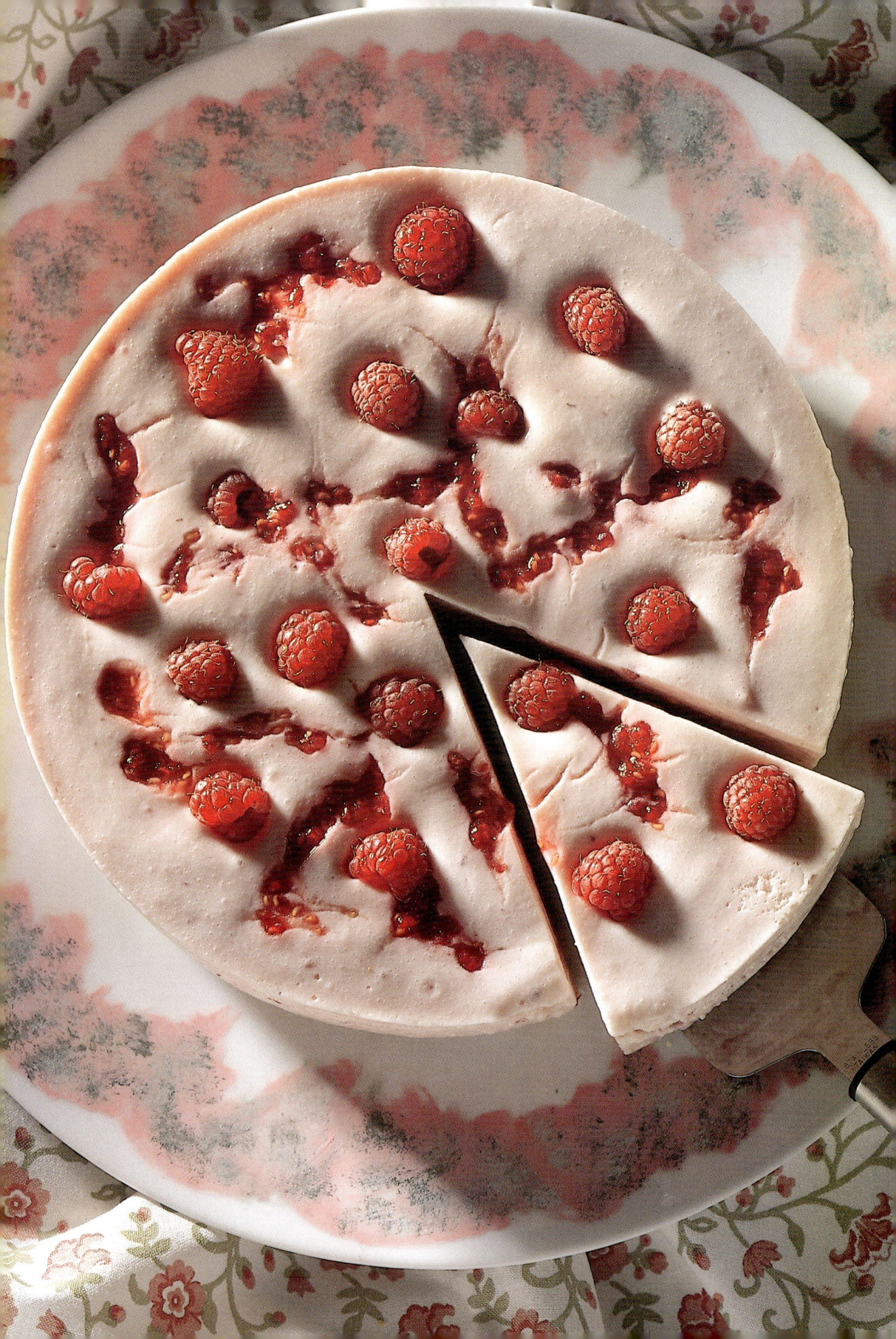

Coconut Rice with Apricot Sauce

2¹/₂ cups skim milk

180g short-grain rice

1 teaspoon each vanilla
and coconut essence

1 tablespoon sugar

1 egg, beaten

SAUCE

2 cups apricot nectar

1 tablespoon arrowroot

1 tablespoon water

6 medium apricots

1. Mix the milk, rice, vanilla essence, coconut essence and sugar in an ovenproof dish and cover. Bake in the oven at 180°C for about 1¹/₂ hours until the rice is cooked, stirring occasionally.

2. Stir in the beaten egg and return to the oven for a further 5 minutes.

3. Spoon the rice into four individual moulds and place in the refrigerator to set.

4. To make the sauce, heat the apricot nectar in a saucepan. Blend the arrowroot and water together to make a smooth mix and stir into the nectar. Cook only until thickened. Remove from the heat and set aside to cool.

5. Invert the rice moulds onto serving plates and garnish each with a quarter of the sauce and the apricots.

SERVES 4

EACH SERVE PROVIDES:
1¹/₂ Fruit, 1¹/₂ Bread, ¹/₂ Milk,
270 Optional Kilojoules.
PER SERVE:
2g Fat, 3g Dietary Fibre.

Sweet Cheese Pancakes

120g plain flour

1 egg

1¼ cups skim milk

1 teaspoon
grated lemon rind

Mint to garnish

FILLING

120g cottage cheese

½ cup fresh or
frozen blueberries

1 tablespoon honey

Drop vanilla essence

SAUCE

1½ cups fresh or
frozen blueberries

1 cup natural
low-fat yoghurt

1. Sift the flour into a bowl and make a well in the centre.

2. In a bowl beat the egg, milk and lemon rind together .

3. Pour this mixture into the well and beat to make a smooth batter. Leave for 30 minutes.

4. Heat a non-stick frying pan and pour in a quarter of the batter to make a large pancake. When the surface becomes dry and bubbles appear, turn the pancake over and cook on the other side for about 1 minute. Leave on a cake rack while cooking the remaining mixture.

5. To prepare the filling, blend or process the cottage cheese, fruit, honey and vanilla essence.

6. In a food processor or blender process the sauce ingredients until smooth. Add artificial sweetener if desired.

7. Place a quarter of the filling in each pancake, roll up and serve with a quarter of the sauce. Garnish with fresh herbs such as mint.

Variation

▶ Raspberries can be used instead of blueberries. Reduce Fruit Selection to ½.

SERVES 4

Each serve provides:
1 Fruit, ¾ Protein,
1½ Bread, ¾ Milk,
125 Optional Kilojoules.
Per serve:
5g Fat, 3g Dietary Fibre.

SNACKS & LUNCHES

Looking for something to snack on or nibble while entertaining friends can often be difficult. In this chapter you will find muffins, dips and drinks to whip up, and all are delicious and healthy at the same time. Lunches can be more than a boring sandwich by using the many types of specialty breads available. Foccacia and pita breads lend themselves to a variety of tasty fillings. Try these snacks and light lunches, which will provide a boost to your day.

Cheese and Ham Muffins

200g plain flour

1 tablespoon baking powder

Pinch salt

60g oat bran

140g grated Cheddar cheese

120g shredded ham

¼ cup minced spring onions

1 egg

1 teaspoon wholegrain mustard

1 cup skim milk

1. Sift the flour, baking powder, salt and oat bran into a bowl. Stir through 120g of the cheese, all the ham and the spring onions. Make a well in the centre.

2. In a jug or bowl, beat the egg, mustard and milk.

3. Using a slotted spoon, fold the liquid ingredients into the dry until just blended. Do not overmix or the muffins will be tough.

4. Spoon the mixture evenly into non-stick muffin pans, making 12 muffins. Top with the remaining cheese.

5. Bake at 200°C for 15 minutes until lightly browned and springy to the touch.

6. Remove from the oven and leave in the pans for 2 to 3 minutes before transferring to a cake rack. Serve warm.

MAKES 12

SERVES OF 1 MUFFIN EACH.
EACH SERVE PROVIDES:
1 Protein, 1 Bread,
35 Optional Kilojoules.
PER SERVE:
5g Fat, 1½g Dietary Fibre.

Left to right; Cheese and Ham Muffins;
Banana and Date Muffins (page 113);
Blueberry Muffins (page 112);
Fruit Drinks (page 120).

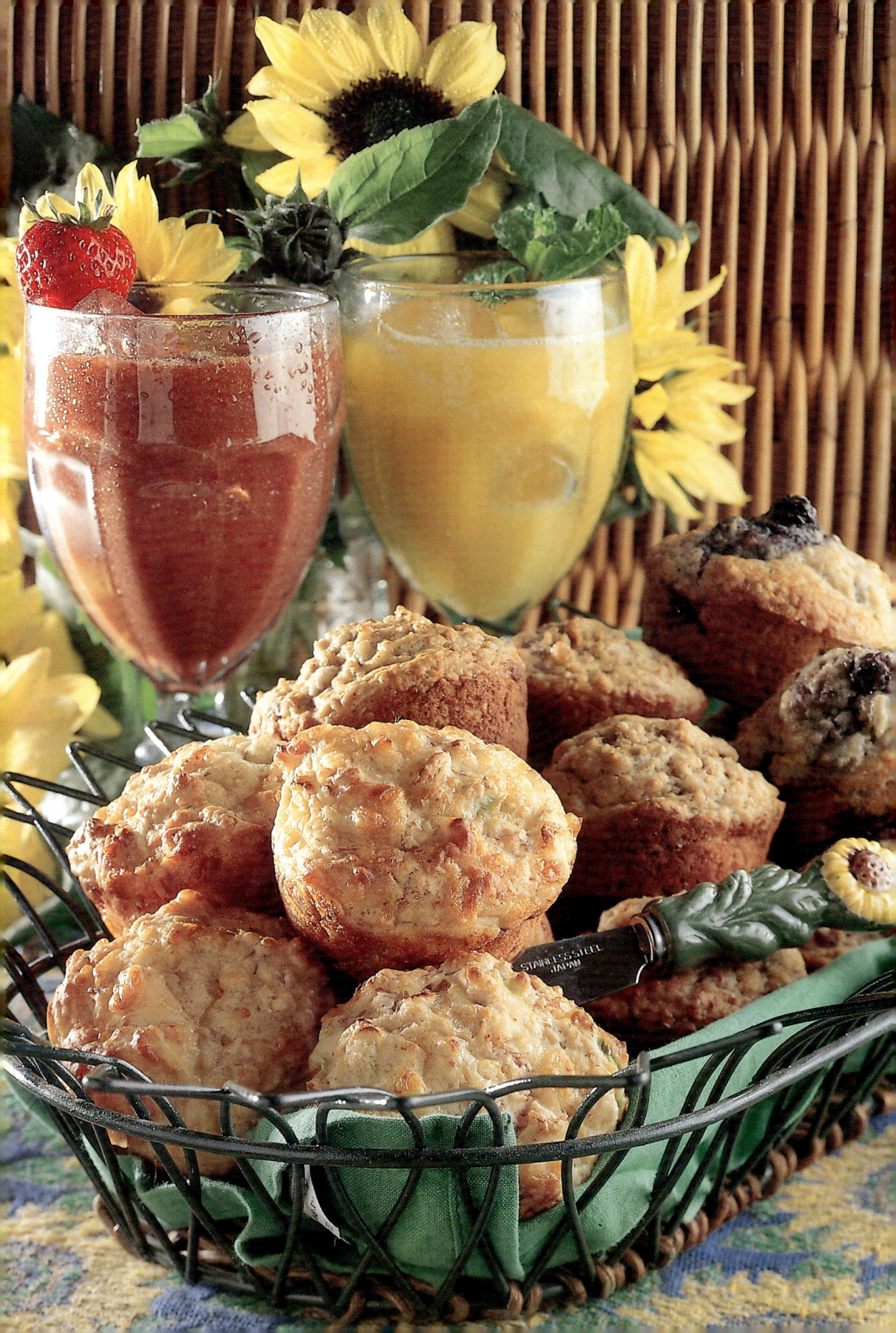

Blueberry Muffins

200g plain flour

1 tablespoon baking powder

1 teaspoon cinnamon

Pinch salt

60g oat bran

1½ tablespoons sugar

60g polyunsaturated margarine, melted

1 cup skim milk

1 egg

2 cups blueberries

1. Sift the flour, baking powder, cinnamon and salt into a bowl. Stir in the oat bran and sugar, and make a well in the centre of the mixture.

2. In another bowl, mix the melted margarine, milk and egg.

3. Using a slotted spoon, fold the liquid ingredients into the dry until just blended. Do not overmix or the muffins will be tough. Add the blueberries.

4. Spoon the mixture evenly into non-stick muffin pans, making 12 muffins.

5. Bake at 200°C for 12 to 15 minutes until lightly browned and springy to touch.

6. Remove from the oven and leave in the pans for 2 to 3 minutes before transferring to a cake rack. Serve warm.

MAKES 12

SERVES OF 1 MUFFIN EACH.
EACH SERVE PROVIDES:
1 Fat, 1 Bread,
150 Optional Kilojoules.
PER SERVE:
5g Fat, 2g Dietary Fibre.

Pictured page 111.

Banana and Date Muffins

200 g plain flour

Pinch salt

$^1/_2$ teaspoon each ground cinnamon and ginger

$^1/_2$ teaspoon baking soda (bicarbonate of soda)

2 teaspoons baking powder

60g oat bran

$1^1/_2$ tablespoons sugar

60g polyunsaturated margarine, melted

1 egg

1 cup buttermilk

2 large bananas, mashed

16 dates, chopped

1. Sift the flour, salt, spices, baking soda and powder into a bowl. Stir in the oat bran and sugar, and make a well in the centre of the mixture.

2. In another bowl, mix the melted margarine, egg, buttermilk, bananas and dates.

3. Using a slotted spoon, fold the liquid ingredients into the dry until just blended. Do not overmix or the muffins will be tough.

4. Spoon the mixture evenly into non-stick muffin pans, making 12 muffins.

5. Bake at 200°C for about 15 to 18 minutes until lightly browned and springy to the touch.

6. Remove from the oven and leave in the pans for 2 to 3 minutes before transferring to a cake rack. Serve warm.

MAKES 12

SERVES OF 1 MUFFIN EACH.
EACH SERVE PROVIDES:
1 Fruit, 1 Fat, 1 Bread,
110 Optional Kilojoules.
PER SERVE:
$5^1/_2$g Fat, 3g Dietary Fibre.

Pictured page 111.

Mushroom Pâté

1 teaspoon olive oil

¹/₂ cup finely chopped onion

2 cups finely sliced mushrooms

¹/₂ cup chicken stock

120g ricotta or cottage cheese

2 tablespoons chopped fresh chervil or parsley

¹/₂ teaspoon black pepper

¹/₂ teaspoon mild mustard

1. Heat the oil in a pan and cook the onion until soft but not brown. Add the mushrooms and cook gently for about 10 minutes until soft.

2. Stir in the chicken stock and simmer for 10 minutes. Set aside to cool.

3. Blend or process the mixture with the ricotta and chervil until smooth.

4. Season well with pepper and mustard, and spoon into four small decorative pâté dishes. Makes about 1 cup.

Cook's Tip

▶ Try serving with Pita Bread Toasts (page 116) or Crostini (30g of each = 1 Bread Selection).

CROSTINI

▶ Slice a French bread stick into 0.5cm thick slices. Place on a baking tray and bake at 180°C until golden and crisp. Serve as a base for a topping or for dipping.

▶ Top crostini with grilled and peeled red capsicum drizzled with cider vinegar and chopped fresh basil (see opposite).

SERVES 4

EACH SERVE PROVIDES:
¹/₂ Protein, 1¹/₄ Vegetable
55 Optional Kilojoules.
PER SERVE:
4¹/₂g Fat, 1g Dietary Fibre.

Snacks from top: Mushroom Pâté; Crostini topped with grilled red capsicum and basil; Hummus on cucumber slices (page 116); grilled eggplant and tomato dippers (page 123); Pita Bread Toasts (page 116).

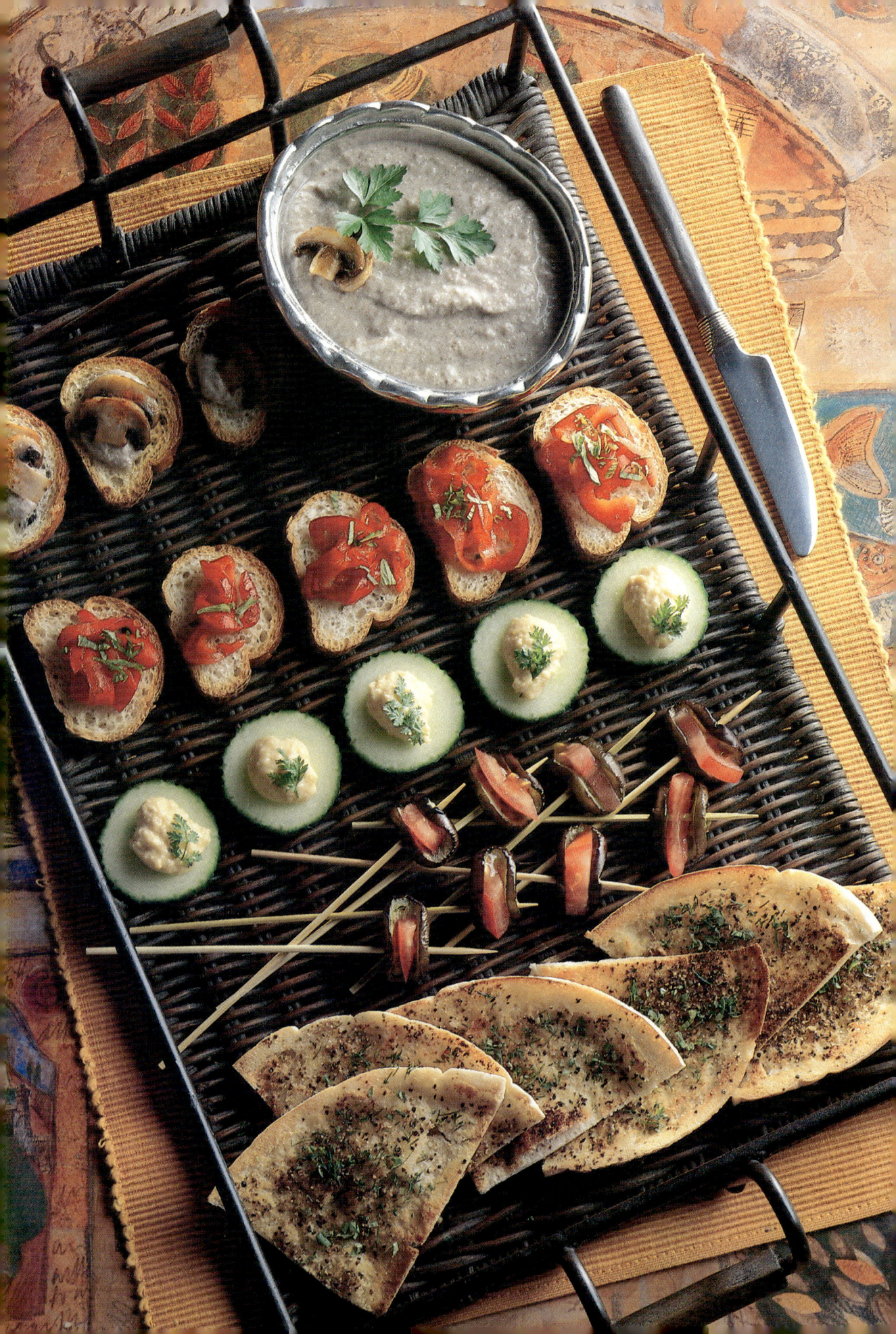

Hummus

180g cooked chick peas

2 tablespoons tahini

2 cloves garlic, peeled

1 teaspoon ground cumin

Pinch ground coriander

2 tablespoons lemon juice

Pinch salt (optional)

1. Blend or process the chick peas, tahini, garlic, cumin, coriander and lemon juice.

2. Season with a pinch of salt if desired.

Cook's Tip

▶ Serve with Crostini (page 114) or Pita Bread Toasts (30g of each = 1 Bread Selection) or slices of cucumber topped with fresh parsley (pictured page 115).

▶ Use as a dip with crisp vegetable sticks.

PITA BREAD TOASTS

▶ Slice the pita breads in half. Melt 1 teaspoon margarine to every 30g bread. Spread the margarine inside the pita breads. Sprinkle with lemon pepper and grill under a moderate heat until crisp (pictured page 115). A good substitute for chips.

▶ Use other flavourings too, such as garlic powder, garlic salt or Cajun sprinkle; or add chopped mixed fresh herbs and black pepper just after grilling and before serving. Pita Bread Toasts store well in an airtight container (30g = 1 Bread Selection. Add 1 Fat to this if you have spread the bread with margarine).

SERVES 4

EACH SERVE PROVIDES:
$^1/_2$ Fat, $^1/_2$ Protein,
$^3/_4$ Bread.
PER SERVE:
$8^1/_2$g Fat, 4g Dietary Fibre.

Savoury Pikelets

¹/₂ cup each grated
zucchini and carrot

1 tablespoon chopped
fresh dill or other herbs

160g self-raising flour

1 cup skim milk

1 egg

1 teaspoon mild mustard

1. Put the vegetables on a microwave-safe plate and cover. Cook on 100% power for 3 to 4 minutes. Alternatively, steam until cooked. Cool and mix in the herbs.

2. Sift the flour into a bowl and toss through the vegetables.

3. Blend the milk, egg and mustard and stir into the floured vegetables. Mix only until combined.

4. Spoon tablespoonfuls onto a pre-heated non-stick pan and cook until bubbles appear on the top. Turn and cook until golden brown.

5. Stack on a cake rack to cool while cooking the remaining pikelets. Serve warm.

Cook's Tip

▶ This recipe transforms the basic pikelet with the addition of a variety of vegetables and herbs. Serve warm with an avocado topping made from blending ¹/₈ avocado with 25mL light sour cream (add ¹/₄ Fat Selection and 50 Optional Kilojoules per serve).

SERVES 4

EACH SERVE PROVIDES:
¹/₂ Vegetable, ¹/₄ Protein
¹/₄ Milk, 2 Bread.
PER SERVE:
2g Fat, 2g Dietary Fibre.

Tabbouli

¹/₂ cup fresh lemon juice

1¹/₂ cups water

180g burghul wheat

1 tablespoon olive oil

1 teaspoon freshly ground black pepper

3 cups chopped ripe tomatoes

¹/₂ cup each chopped fresh Italian parsley and mint

¹/₂ cup chopped onion

¹/₄ cup chopped spring onions

2 garlic cloves, crushed

1. In a saucepan, bring the lemon juice and water to the boil. Add the burghul, oil and pepper. Remove from heat, cover, and let stand 20 to 25 minutes.

2. In a large bowl combine the tomatoes, parsley, mint, onion, spring onions and garlic. Toss well to mix. Add burghul mixture and toss well again.

3. Transfer burghul mixture to a large serving bowl. Refrigerate, covered, for 3 hours until thoroughly chilled.

Cook's Tip

▶ Serve for lunch. Split a pita bread almost in two and place lettuce leaves inside. Fill with tabbouli and diced, cooked lamb, seasoned with pepper.

SERVES 6

EACH SERVE PROVIDES:
1¹/₂ Vegetable, ³/₄ Fat
1¹/₂ Bread.
Per Serve:
3g Fat, 7g Dietary Fibre.

Sandwich ideas: A pita bread pocket filled with lettuce, tabbouli and sliced roast lamb (left) and foccacia bread with sliced tomatoes and mushrooms.

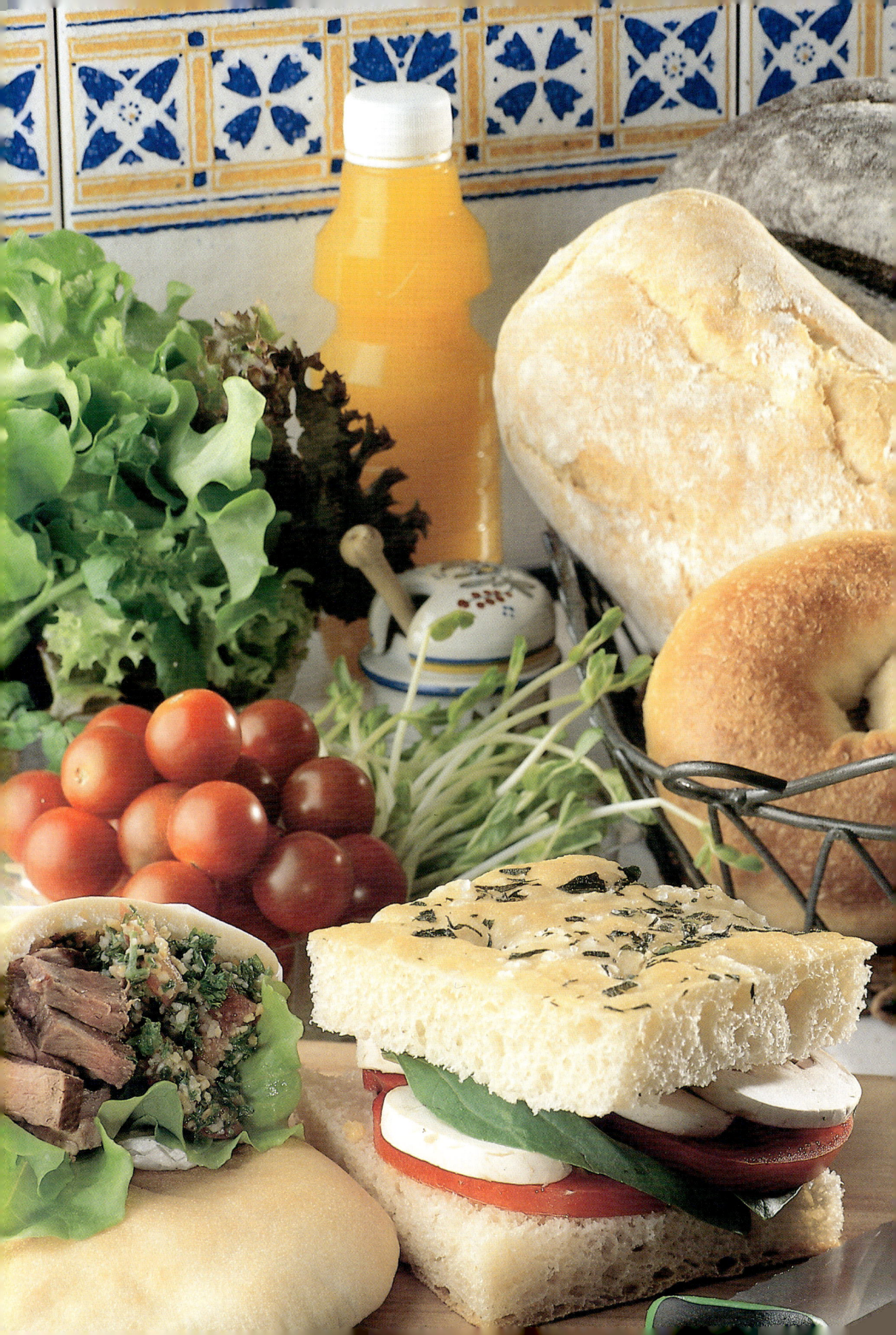

Fruit Drinks

1 ripe peach, sliced

½ cup orange juice

½ cup crushed ice

1. In a food processor or blender, combine the peach slices and orange juice and whizz until smooth.

2. Add the ice and whizz just long enough to ensure the ice remains crunchy.

3. Serve in a tall, chilled glass (pictured page 111).

Variations

▶ ⅓ cup prune juice and ½ cup strawberries. Blend and serve over crushed ice (pictured page 111). Each serve provides: 1½ Fruit. Per serve: 0g Fat, 8g Dietary Fibre.

▶ 1 small apple, 2 tablespoons lemon juice and ½ cup apple juice. Blend all ingredients until smooth and serve well chilled. Each serve provides: 2 Fruit. Per serve: 0g Fat, 3g Dietary Fibre.

▶ ½ cup orange juice, the pulp of 3 passionfruit and ½ cup crushed ice. Whiz. Each serve provides: 2 Fruit. Per serve: ½g Fat, 13g Dietary Fibre.

▶ 1 cup diced watermelon, ½ cup crushed ice and a few fresh mint sprigs. Blend and serve in a tall glass. Each serve provides: 1 Fruit. Per serve: ½g Fat, 1g Dietary Fibre.

▶ 1 cup raspberries and ½ cup orange juice. Blend and serve over crushed ice. Each serve provides: 2 Fruit. Per serve: 0g Fat, 10g Dietary Fibre.

Cook's Tip

▶ Remember to keep a packet of frozen berries in the freezer during the winter months. When the shelves are quite lean, frozen fruit can add variety.

SERVES 1

EACH SERVE PROVIDES:
2 Fruit.
PER SERVE:
0g Fat, 1½ Dietary Fibre.

Milk Shakes

1 cup skim milk

¹/₂ small banana, sliced

¹/₂ cup blackberries

¹/₂ cup ice cubes

1. In a food processor or blender, combine the milk, banana slices, blackberries and ice and whip until the mixture is thick and frothy.

2. Serve in a tall, chilled glass.

Variations

Mix two half fruit serves together for more variety. Try one of these combinations:

▶ Peaches and raspberries.

▶ Strawberries and plums.

▶ Pineapple and dried apricots.

▶ Mango and orange.

▶ Passionfruit pulp and pawpaw.

▶ Apricots and a few drops of coconut essence.

Cook's Tip

▶ Mix half a yoghurt serve and half a milk serve together. It will result in a thick tangy shake which you can vary by using different flavoured low-fat yoghurt. Add the fruit of your choice.

SERVES 1

EACH SERVE PROVIDES:
1 Fruit, 1 Milk.
PER SERVE:
¹/₂ g Fat, 2¹/₂ Dietary Fibre.

Snack Attack

SERVES 2

EACH SERVE PROVIDES:
1 Bread, 2 Fruit.
PER SERVE:
4g Fat, 5g Dietary Fibre.

POPCORN

▶ Pop the corn in the microwave and mix with chopped dried fruits. For example, 2 cups popcorn with 6 dried apricot halves, chopped, and 20g sultanas.

Variation

▶ Instead of fruit, toss in spicy flavourings such as lemon and pepper, Cajun, Italian or Mexican flavoured sprinkles.

SERVES 2

EACH SERVE PROVIDES:
1 Fat, 1 Protein or Bread.
PER SERVE:
6g Fat, 3g Dietary Fibre.

CHICK PEA SNACK

▶ Mix 120g cooked chick peas with $1/2$ teaspoon each curry powder and turmeric, and toss in 2 teaspoons vegetable oil. Roast at 180°C for 35–40 minutes until well cooked.

Cook's Tip

▶ Make up two to three times this quantity, store in an airtight container and use as required.

SERVES 1

EACH SERVE PROVIDES:
1 Fruit, $1/2$ Protein, 1 Bread.
PER SERVE:
5g Fat, 6g Dietary Fibre.

FRUIT SLICES

▶ Take a slice of fruit loaf or half a fruit bread muffin and top it with 30g ricotta cheese and one serving of fruit, such as 6 apricot halves, sliced; 20g diced figs or prunes; or half a mango, sliced.

Cook's Tip

▶ Try toasting the fruit bread, for a change.

Dips

To prepare dips, combine the ingredients of your choice to form a smooth dip. Try the following suggestions:

▶ Boil a 400g can of savoury tomatoes down to ½ cup, until thick and pulpy. Flavour with fresh herbs. Use as a dip with vegetables sticks.

▶ Mix light sour cream with natural low-fat plain yoghurt, plenty of mixed herbs, a dash of minced garlic, salt and pepper.

▶ Blend equal quantities of ricotta cheese and feta cheese, and flavour with garlic and a few chopped olives. Smooth with milk to make a dipping consistency.

▶ Make a thick cheese sauce and cool. Spice it up with Mexican flavours such as fresh coriander and jalepeño peppers. Serve warm as a dipping sauce.

▶ Combine natural low-fat yoghurt and plenty of chopped fresh mint. It's an easy one to make up in advance!

DUNKERS

Use one of the bread suggestions below, remembering that 30g = 1 Bread Selection. If you use margarine, add 1 Fat Selection.

▶ Crostini or Pita Bread Toasts (see pages 114 and 116).

▶ Grilled thin slices of eggplant and tomato on skewers (pictured page 115).

CRUDITÉS

Crudités are crisp vegetable dunkers and are delicious when fresh. Add them to your snack list. You can assess how many crudités make ½ cup vegetables or 1 serve, so you can calculate your daily intake. Keep the vegetables in an airtight container in the fridge. Try some of the following ideas:

▶ Asparagus, peeled with the rough ends trimmed and blanched.

▶ Brussels sprouts, trimmed and halved.

▶ Carrots, peeled and cut into sticks.

▶ Cauliflower and broccoli florets.

▶ Celery, cut into sticks.

▶ Cucumber, deseeded and cut into sticks.

▶ Green beans, stringed and blanched.

▶ Radishes, trimmed and whole or halved.

▶ Tomatoes, whole cherry tomatoes or quartered tomatoes.

▶ Zucchini, trimmed and cut into sticks.

Sandwich Fillings

For lunch try any of these delicious filling ideas with one of the different styles of bread available such as foccacia or pita bread.

VEGETABLE IDEAS
- ▶ Grated fresh beetroot with dill and mung bean sprouts.
- ▶ Fresh spinach, bean sprouts and fresh parsley.
- ▶ Sliced cold potatoes, fresh mint, ham and lettuce.
- ▶ Grated carrot, peanut butter and orange.
- ▶ Sliced mushrooms, red capsicum, spinach and spring onions.
- ▶ Chopped hard-cooked egg, snow pea sprouts, blanched snow peas and lettuce.
- ▶ Tomatoes and mushrooms, sliced, and fresh basil.

WITH CHEESE
- ▶ Ricotta cheese with minced celery, green capsicum and a spicy pickle.
- ▶ Crushed pineapple, grated Cheddar cheese, spring onions and fresh mint.
- ▶ Cottage cheese, Vegemite and lettuce leaves.
- ▶ Chopped gherkins, grated hard cheese and a few capers.
- ▶ Cottage cheese, chopped dates and grated lemon or orange rind.

WITH MEAT
- ▶ Lean roast beef and horseradish sauce or sliced canned artichokes and pickle.
- ▶ Smoked chicken, grated swede and carrot and chopped fresh parsley.
- ▶ Diced chicken, pineapple or mango, chopped fresh mint, diced capsicum and a tablespoon of cottage or ricotta cheese.
- ▶ Sliced surimi, lettuce, fresh pawpaw and chilli sauce.
- ▶ Tuna, lettuce, sliced radishes and chopped olives.
- ▶ Canned salmon, sliced fresh tomatoes and fresh basil.
- ▶ Slices of rare roast beef, sliced fresh apples or pears, mild mustard and a few mung bean sprouts.
- ▶ Shaved ham or cold pork, dates and pineapple.
- ▶ Diced lean lamb, cooked eggplant, lettuce, mint and yoghurt.

TOASTED SANDWICH FILLINGS
- ▶ Banana, mashed with ham and cheese.
- ▶ Baked beans and cheese.
- ▶ Cottage cheese, raisins and pineapple.

NOTE: Check Program for serving information.

Glossary

Arrowroot: Used for thickening; cornflour can be substituted.

Bean Sprouts: Also known as bean shoots.

Bicarbonate of Soda: Baking soda.

Blanch: To partly cook vegetables for a short time so they need little or no further cooking.

Bok Choy (Chinese white cabbage): Remove and discard stems, use leaves and young tender parts of stems.

Burghul (cracked wheat): Wheat that is steamed until partly cooked, then dried and cracked.

Capers: Pickled flower buds from a Mediterranean shrub.

Capsicum: Peppers, red or green.

Cardamom: Spice with an exotic fragrance, available in pod, seed or ground form.

Castor Sugar: Fine white granulated sugar.

Cheese:

Brie: Soft French cheese.

Feta: Very salty white Greek cheese, cured in brine.

Parmesan: Sharp-tasting hard cheese used to flavour.

Quark: A low-fat cheese.

Ricotta: Soft white Italian dessert cheese.

Chick Peas: Also known as garbanzos, when canned. Dried peas need to be soaked, preferably overnight.

Coriander: Strongly flavoured herb also known as cilantro or Chinese parsley.

Couscous: A finely ground cereal made from semolina.

Dash: Less than $1/8$ teaspoon of an ingredient.

Eggplant: Aubergine.

Fennel: Has an aniseed taste. While the bulb and fronds are used, seeds are also ground as a component of curry powder.

Filo Pastry: Tissue-thin pastry sheets bought chilled or frozen.

Five Spice Powder: A combination of cinnamon, star anise, cloves, fennel and Szechwan peppers, often used in Chinese cooking.

Flake: To break food into flat pieces, usually with a fork.

Flour: Use plain or all-purpose flour unless otherwise stated.

Gelatine: A setting agent.

Ginger: Fresh, root or green ginger; scrape away outside skin and grate, chop or slice as required.

Hoisin Sauce: Thick, sweet Chinese sauce made from salted black beans, onions and garlic.

Indonesian Soy Sauce (Kepjap Manis): Soy sauce sweetened with palm sugar.

Jalapeño Peppers: Imported, canned, pickled, hot chillies.

Leeks: Member of the onion family, resembles the spring onion but is much larger. Use only the white part unless the recipe states otherwise.

Lemon Grass: Available fresh, dried or canned. Fresh must be bruised or chopped before using to release flavour.

Lentils: There are many different types of lentils; some require overnight soaking.

Lettuce:

Butter: Soft texture with a flat, smooth leaf and a mild flavour.

Cos: Also known as Romaine, has coarse, dark green leaves which are crunchy and slightly astringent.

Curly Endive: Long, lacy leaves, mildly bitter in flavour.

Iceberg: The most common variety, has a large heart, is sweet-flavoured and stays crisp.

Mignonette: Soft, small leaves with red tinge and slightly bitter.

Radicchio: Type of Italian lettuce with dark burgundy leaves and a slightly bitter taste.

Rocket: Also known as Aragula, with small dark green leaves and a strong, peppery flavour.

Naan Bread: An Indian leavened bread, traditionally made in a Tandoor or clay oven.

Nashi: A fruit, flavoured like a pear with the crispness of an apple.

Pappadums: Thin, crisp Indian wafer bread, made from rice flour or spiced potato.

Pawpaw: Papaya.

Pita Bread: Flat bread with a pocket in the centre.

Rice:

Arborio: From Italy, a large round-grained rice used for risotto.

Basmati: Similar appearance to long grain white rice; aromatic with a firm texture.

Brown: Natural whole-grain; takes longer to cook than white rice.

Jasmine: Thai long grain rice, mildly fragrant.

White: Hulled and polished, can be short or long grained.

Sesame Oil: Extracted from sesame seeds, this has a strong nutty flavour.

Simmer: To cook in liquid just below the boiling point.

Snow Peas: Also known as mange tout, sugar peas or Chinese peas.

Soy Sauce: Made from fermented soy beans; we used the low-salt variety.

Spinach, English: Soft-leaved vegetable, more delicate in taste than silverbeet; however, young silverbeet can be substituted.

Spring Onions: Known as shallots or green onions in some Australian states; scallions in some other countries.

Surimi: Imitation crab meat.

Sweet Potatoes: Kumara.

Tofu: Firm, soft and silken textures are available. Also known as bean curd.

Tomato:

Tomato Paste: A concentrated tomato purée used in flavouring soups, stews, sauces etc.

Tomato Purée: Canned, puréed tomatoes; use fresh, peeled, puréed tomatoes as a substitute.

Sun-dried: Dried tomatoes, often bottled in oil.

Vermicelli: Thin Italian egg noodles.

Water Chestnuts: Dark brown tubers which are peeled to reveal white flesh. Available canned.

White Fish: Non-oily varieties, including John Dory, bream, flathead, whiting, snapper, jew–fish and ling.

Wontons: Thin pastry sold fresh or frozen, used in Chinese cooking for stuffing.

Zucchini: Courgette.

Index